Social and Historical Foundations of Modern Medicine

By

IAGO GALDSTON, M.D.

BRUNNER/MAZEL, Publishers • New York

Library of Congress Cataloging in Publication Data

Galdston, Iago, 1895-
Social and historical foundations of modern medicine.

Includes bibliographical references and index.
1. Medicine—History. 2. Social medicine—History. I. Title.
[DNLM: 1. History of medicine. WZ 40 G149s]
R131.G26 362.1'09 81-1896

ISBN 0-87630-259-2 AACR2

Published by
BRUNNER/MAZEL, INC.
19 Union Square
New York, New York 10003

MANUFACTURED IN THE UNITED STATES OF AMERICA

TO THE MEMORIES OF

JOHN A. RYLE

HENRY E. SIGERIST

LORD COHEN OF BIRKENHEAD

Foreword

Among physicians, a taste for medical history commonly appears late in life. So long as one need not live there, the past makes an agreeable change from the present; and the part-time historian's chance of making some small discovery is greater than that of the part-time golfer or gardener.

What he discovers is sometimes interesting in itself; and to add to any kind of knowledge is fun. Nevertheless, to me, at least, medical history seems no more than a pleasant pastime, unless its findings can be shown to bear on what we are doing today. Or not doing.

Dr. Galdston is neither a dilettante who flirts with medical history, nor a professional who is wedded to it. Instead, he has been, for forty years and more, a devoted amateur whose concern has arisen out of his labours as a clinician. What distinguishes him among students of the past is that he cares less about *Who?* and *What?* and *Where?* than about *Why?*

The common belief that Medicine has advanced continuously and triumphantly, from Hippocrates to the present day, he finds ill founded. On the contrary, its progress has been episodic, depending largely on extraneous factors—mostly economic and cultural.

One big cultural change is that to the agrarian Greek, and their successors, man was part of Nature; living with it, not outside it; but when science erupted in the 16th and 17th century, this ecological view was abandoned. By taking thought, it was now felt, man could make himself master of the Universe; and in this glorious pursuit, everything became expendable, including human life and happiness. Whatever progress might cost, it was deemed a bargain.

And so man became, in Dr. Galdston's words, "The wastrel of the earth." Believing that, in time, he will be able to do anything whatever, he shows himself "an ecologic ignoramus." After all, it is only to himself that he is the pinnacle of Creation.

Medicine, of course, has benefited immensely from the sciences. But it is not itself a science, for its search for truth is secondary to its care of human beings.

The proper care of human beings should include promotion of their health; and, "Health," as Dr. Galdston says, "means more than the absence of disease." Medicine, therefore, should stop thinking almost solely in terms of disease; and, great though its achievements are, they could be even greater if it jettisoned the idea that all we have to deal with is an array of specific diseases, for each of which a specific remedy can eventually be found.

Admittedly, in countering epidemic and endemic infections and infestations, the "specific" approach has had wonderful victories. But we are now entering a period in which the "disorders of faulty existence" have come into the foreground—especially, in developed countries. In their incidence and distribution, coronary disease, hypertension, peptic ulcer, and diabetes do not behave like tuberculosis or measles. Nor do alcoholism, divorce, suicide, schizophrenia, and the "psychosomatic" disturbances that nowadays confront the physician so often. Approaches useful in one setting are inappropriate in another; and in few, if any, of these disorders can we reasonably hope to find a single specific means of cure—a "magic bullet."

Medicine, in fact, took a wrong turning when concentration on disease began to distract attention from the person diseased.

For those who, too simply, see our task as the conquest of specific diseases, diagnosis is no more than the process of distinguishing one from another—a process which the laboratory is nowadays taking over. For Dr. Galdston, needless to say, diagnosis is, or should be, something more comprehensive: "The summation of all that deviates from the normal in a sick individual of definite psychological and physical endowments living under particular circumstances in a given milieu." Even a computerized laboratory is hardly capable of this!

With so broad a view, Dr. Galdston is, naturally, impatient with the narrowness of medical education; and he urges, in effect, that the student's teaching should be based on human ecology rather than nosology.

Whatever its basis, it must, of course, be practical too. All through the ages, the man with a dislocated shoulder has wanted the same thing—somebody who will restore the joint as quickly and painlessly as possible. Sometimes, the local bonesetter, fetched from the smithy, was, at least, as successful as a modern graduate, and much more expeditious than most hospital teams. Moreover, instead of sending a bill, he might be content with a couple of rabbits for his supper.

Dr. Galdston would, I am sure, agree that, however well students are taught about social medicine, or about homeostasis, many of them will still be interested chiefly in how to put a shoulder right, and in the skillful use of the innumerable drugs now at their command. Many of them will always be pragmatists, more at home with practice than with theory; for which, we should probably be thankful. But my mention of the village bonesetter illustrates another, and more important, point made over and over again in these pages. History shows that efficient medical care can be given by many different kinds of people, in many different circumstances. So we should not suppose that there are no alternatives to the present patterns of medical practice; or that the sacredness of our favorite cows has been certified for all eternity.

Like many of the rest of us, Dr. Galdston finds the present patterns neither wholly suitable nor wholly effective; and he wants the emphasis shifted towards physiological medicine and public health—the first concerned with man's internal milieu, the second with his external.

Perhaps he is right in regarding some of his ideas as revolutionary; for he challenges much that most people take for granted; for example, that disease can be conquered. But his book is not one that pursues an argument, relentlessly, to some controversial end. Like progress, it is discontinuous—a collection of papers to be read in any order, leaving the reader to choose his subjects and reach his own conclusions.

Because the papers were mostly prepared for fellow historians, parts of some of them are caviar to the general. But his writing can be so vivid, and forceful, and witty, that even the abstruse may be absorbing. At least one essay deserves a place in a literary anthology—if only as an elegant diatribe.

Apart from the pleasure of reading them, do his reflections matter? Unquestionably, yes; because he has things to say that really do throw light on what is going on now. By the increase of automation, and the like, our society is being speedily transformed; and Dr. Galdston is all too right in fearing that, "The values which man has lived by and prized, those of diligent work, of thrift, of individual initiative, of charity, of mutual aid, of intimate shared responsibilities within the family and beyond in the community—all these and others beside will be rendered nugatory." More and more, man is being "denatured," and the result is likely to be "personal and political alienation and a pervasive sense of seemingly purposeless lives." Against this, it is encouraging that the threat is widely recognized. "No previous age facing a truly radical technological innovation attained to a similar awareness of challenge and menace."

For our loss of nerve, where there is one, Dr. Galdston's remedy is a return to humanism—faith in man, hope in man, and charity towards man; yet, with no illusions about him. We must have "large perspectives, willingness to wait for results, competence to endure, intelligence to recognize divergences, and profound faith in the educability of man."

In Medicine, he believes, our accustomed orientations will no longer serve. "To set things aright, we need not only to learn much that is new, but also to unlearn much that is old and in error." We have been acquiring wrong attitudes towards disease and towards health; and we should think again.

Those of us, that is, with time enough ahead to change the future!

Sir Theodore Fox
Former Editor
of the British *Lancet*

Contents

Acknowledgments

The pursuit of the studies presented in this volume has been exciting, exacting, inspiring and rewarding. The yields appear to me to be even more timely now than they were when first gained.

I cannot pay my respects and thanks to more than a fraction of those who have helped me, for these studies extended for more than forty years. Foremost among them I count Henry Sigerist, first professor of medical history at The Johns Hopkins University. Cro-magnon in appearance, Renaissance in spirit, erudite in the classical sense, he was teacher, friend and counselor to me. I pay warm tribute to his memory.

A less intimate but equally fruitful association was with Dr. John Alfred Ryle, who in 1943 resigned his chair as Regius Professor of Physics at Cambridge to initiate the study of social medicine at Oxford. To Lord Horder and Lord Cohen of Birkenhead, both leaders in British medicine, I am deeply in debt for their help and encouragement. I owe a similar debt to Dr. James Macalister Mackintosh, Dean of the London School of Hygiene and Tropical Medicine. The Commonwealth Fund, under the directorship of Mr. Barry Smith, and the Milbank Memorial Foundation, with Dr. Frank Boudreau as its Director, generously supported my studies with sundry grants. The NIMH also favored me with a grant for study of the development and history of medical education.

In their original form these essays appeared in the following Journals: *Bulletin of the New York Academy of Medicine* (Prometheus and the Gods, Trade Routes and Medicine, The Epidemic Constitution); *Bulletin of the History of Medicine* (Diagnosis in Historical Perspective, Social Medicine and the Epidemic Constitution, Historical Epochs in Medical Education); *The Journal of the Wellcome Institute of the History of Medicine* (Medicine and Culture, The Pathogenicity of Progress); *The Wenner-Gren Foundation of Anthropological and Ethnological Research* (Technology, Culture and Disease); *The Journal of Medical Education*

(Doctor and Patient in Medical History); *The Yale Journal of Biology and Medicine* (The Amateur in Medical History); *The Canadian Medical Association Journal* (On the Futility of Medical History); *Journal of the American Medical Association* (The Birth and Death of Specialties); *Annals of Medical History* (Humanism and Public Health). I am indebted to the Editors of these journals for permission to republish.

SOCIAL AND HISTORICAL FOUNDATIONS OF MODERN MEDICINE

1

Medicine and Culture

To the best of my knowledge, admittedly neither global nor encyclopaedic, no historian of medicine has ever composed a history of medicine in which cultural factors are presented as major determinants. Sigerist, had he lived long enough and continued to write, would perhaps have authored such a work. In his later years he had become astutely aware of the extent to which political, economic, and technological conditions influence the directions of development in medicine.

To study the medicine of different cultures is by no means the same as studying the relationship between culture and medicine. Every "standard" history of medicine begins with some chapters on primitive medicine, Mesopotamian medicine, Egyptian medicine, the medicine of the Hebrews, the Greeks, the Romans, et al. These chapters give, to the extent they do, the history of distinctive peoples possessed (or so it is assumed) of distinctive cultures and of medical ideas and practices differing from those of other peoples. Such chapters are not devoted to an exposition of how the cultural realities and characteristics of the given people shaped its medicine and were conversely influenced. They are merely descriptive, though not infrequently judgmental in an open or covert manner. "The doctors of the period believed in spells, talismans, astrology; they were ignorant, superstitious, and most probably frauds," and so forth.

This is perhaps overdrawn as a generalization, but it is sufficiently representative of the predominant persuasion to call for no radical conditioning. I recall few instances in which medical historians have attempted to expound the dynamic interrelations of a given culture with its unique medical theories and practices. Why the overspecialization in Egyptian medicine? Why the four humours of Greek medicine? Why the rejection of Galenic medicine so late? Why the *Contagium vivum*—so late in history? Why the modern concept of specificity?

Medical historians, the rare exceptions granted, have not occupied themselves with such questions. In fact, any question beginning with or containing the word *why* is anathema to the academic historian of medicine. The terrain of their interest is bordered by *what, when, where* and *how*. The question *why* generally throws them into a resentful dither, and their stock reaction is to respond, in a testy tone, "The question is unscientific."

Perhaps it is asking too much of the academic medical historians to suggest that he think "in the configurations of cultural anthropology." Historians by and large are not well informed in that area. They are not trained to think anthropologically.

Why then single out the academic medical historians? For positive as well as negative reasons: not only because of what they fail to teach, but also and even more so because of what they do teach.

I will formulate my argument in relation to the medical historiography of the last hundred and fifty years. In its more sophisticated pattern, this commences with "paleopathology." To effectively portray the "progress" of medicine, it is indeed necessary first to emphasize the antiquity of disease; then, by contrast, one can portray the recency of the effective treatment, control, and eradication of disease.

Paleopathology shows by the remains of ancient Man that disorders known to us at the present time also afflicted prehistoric Man. It shows that the modes of the body's reactions to pathogenic agents have not changed during known time. The mummified remains of the Egyptian tuberculous "hunchback" pictured in numerous works touching on the antiquity of disease reveal exactly the same pathological changes as the hunchbacks we ourselves encountered when tuberculosis was still rife. And such findings give rise to the contention that disease is a constant phenomenon, historically unchanged and unchanging, in respect to its causations, pathologies, and symptomatologies.

As much is also said of the pathogens. The tubercle bacilli of antiquity are assumed to have been identical with their present day descendants.

The idea that disease and its causes are constant finds further support in the pharmacodynamic effects of some of the specific remedies employed in ancient times, which are as certain today as they were in the past.

From all this, it is concluded that disease is independent of time and place, and so too, in a measure, are the therapeutic agents. Syphilis, cancer, tuberculosis are the same at the ends of the world. Penicillin is as effective in the United States as in India. Physiological and endocrine disorders have a common, universal, unvarying aetiological basis.

Such instances and examples lead to the belief that while medicine is not as exact a science as is chemistry or physics, it is *au fond* an exact science, becoming increasingly so as more and more of its besetting uncertainties are cleared up. In this view, medical history is the story of the emergence and evolution of medicine from ignorance, superstition and empiricism up to its present state as a scientific discipline.

It is this persuasion that inspires the facile phrase, so reminiscent of the *memento mori* of time past, "Psychiatry is now where medicine was two hundred years ago."

Unquestionably, medicine has made great progress during the past two hundred years, to take an arbitrary period. It has gained enormously in precise knowledge. In many respects, both informationally and technically, it has become more exact.

But that doesn't make it an exact science. Indeed, on close examination, the arguments and deductions based on the antiquity and alleged constancy of disease are found to be of doubtful validity and, where valid, of limited significance. The carious bone of the prehistoric tuberculosis victim demonstrates only, if it demonstrates that much, that the tubercle bacillus lodged in human bone affects with some constancy the noted gross interreactions with the host tissue. The carious bone tells us nothing about how its owner once experienced his disease, how he felt about it, what he attributed it to, how he bore up under it, what his medicine man, shaman, or healer thought about it, how he accounted for its origin, what was the nature and theoretical framework of *his* practice, what his philosophical orientation. It doesn't tell us what other persons thought of the man's disease and how they related to him because of it. In other words, it tells us very little about the disease and nothing at all about *the man who suffered the disease* nor anything else that concerns the man and the world he lived in.

This brings us to face with a crucial question: What is medicine? Is it a science whose subject matter is *'disease, its cause, cure and prevention'*? Or, is it a discipline concerned with man (ill and well) whose living experience invariably and inevitably includes pain, disease and death?

The straddle answer, "It is part of each, or both," is meaningless and evasive. Of course, as a discipline concerned with Man and his life's experience, medicine by definition must also be concerned with disease, its cause, cure, and prevention. But medicine as a science whose subject matter is disease, its cause, cure, and prevention, need not be, and in recent historical experience has become less and less concerned and involved with *the man who is diseased.* How otherwise could clinicians talk in earnest about the computer's coming takeover of medical practice?

Interested as we are in the interrelation of medicine and culture, the question "What is medicine?" must be of prime importance. For if the answer be that it is "a science" of the same order as those labeled *exact sciences*—then we cannot but conclude that it has little relation to culture. If, on the other hand, the answer is that medicine is a humanistic discipline, concerned with Man and his life experiences—a discipline that utilizes the exact sciences but is itself other than, and I would add more than, an exact science—then it follows that medicine must be of the very "web and woof" of culture.

During most of medical history, medicine was deemed a *scientia,* an organized body of knowledge, but not a science, not even a pure *techne* in the Greek sense. Hippocrates referred to medicine as *the Art.* Medicine acquired the pretence of an exact science during the 19th century when the exact sciences, notably physics and chemistry, developed substance and stature. Medicine made its formal declaration of suffrage among the exact sciences in the pronouncement of Du Bois Reymond to the effect that the biological sciences need not and will not acknowledge the operations of any other forces but those of chemistry and physics. Michael Polanyi, in his article *Scientific Outlook: Its Sickness and Cure* (1), reminds us that in 1948 K. S. Lashley reconfirmed Du Bois Reymond's declaration. Addressing a symposium on Cerebral Mechanisms in Behaviour, Lashley declared, "Our common meeting ground is the faith to which we all subscribe, I believe, that the phenomena of behavior and of mind are ultimately describable in the concepts of the physical and mathematical sciences." Polanyi adds: "It is in fact taken almost universally for granted among neurologists, who regard its acceptance as inherent in their claim to be scientists. Yet I," Polanyi affirms, "do not think anybody can hold this belief." Of many penetrating observations in Polanyi's article, I want to borrow one which relates to "detached analysis." "There are," he wrote, "a great number of things our knowledge of which dissolves if we look at them in a thoroughly detached manner" (2). Practiced as a science, medicine detaches the disease from the man who suffers it; in consequence, to use Polanyi's phrase, our knowledge of both dissolves.

During the greater part of historic medicine, there was no such detachment. The disease was not abstracted from the patient, and the patient was not abstracted from the world he lived in nor from Nature itself. "I treat him—Nature cures him," was the protestation of the Greek physician. This dependence of man on Nature was perceived and acknowledged down the ages and is encountered in a somewhat modified version in Paré's words, "I bandage him—God heals him."

In Greek medicine—and Greek medicine in effect prevailed in Europe for close to two thousand years—Man was seen not merely as dependent upon Nature, but as an inseparable part of manifest Nature. In classical Greek culture, the concept of *physis,* of Nature, was central and dominant, and in medicine it afforded the physician a rationale for health and sickness, and a rationale, too, for his therapeutic efforts. Health was the resultant of living in accordance with Nature's requisites; disease the result of the failure to do so. The good physician was one schooled and skilled in diagnosing what was the trouble and whence it came, and in helping Nature by means of the prescribed regimen to reestablish the patient's health.

Greek culture was conditioned by its economy, which was predominantly agrarian. It is understandable, then, why the concept of Nature, of *physis,* was preeminent. It can be said that Hippocrates wrote medicine like an intelligent, observant and experienced farmer. For who better than the farmer can appreciate the function for good or bad of airs, waters, and places? In the Hippocratic theory of the four qualities—hot, cold, moist and dry—one can recognize an astute generalization derived from long agrarian experience. Good soil being given, it is the right balance of the four qualities that favors a bountiful crop. And a bountiful crop favors the well-being of the animal world, man included. Hippocrates was much concerned with food. Like Hesiod before him, he traces the origins of medicine to the observations of what was edible and good for Man and what was not.

It may not be expressed anywhere in so many words, but illness had for the Greeks a connotation of sin. This differed radically from the Christian view that illness was God's punishment of the sinner for his moral transgressions. In fact, Hippocrates maintained in the *Sacred Disease* that a god might purify, but would not defile the human body with sickness.

Yet the concept of physis implies a reciprocal, almost contractual, relation between Man and Nature. It is as if Nature warned, "Follow my ways and you will be well; violate them and you will be ill." Yet Nature was not punitive, for she "willed" to do what she could for the man who was sick, if he would but lend himself, the physician guiding and helping, to her healing efforts. Hence the sick man was a man who had sinned against Nature, and sickness carried with it a moral issue. I underscore this because the element of morality has no place at all in modern-day medicine. There is no sin, moral injustice, or social wrong that is not ultimately explicable and frequently is explained in terms of disease. The physician who is not judgmental is praised and prized.

In the Greek classical writings, madness in large measure was ascribed to the volitional acts of the afflicted. The gods, demons, Erinyes may have entered into the play of destiny, but always it was some individual brash or evil act that sealed the doom.

The Greek physician shied away from undertaking to treat the untreatable. This has been judged by some as a base, craven avoidance of the physician's duty. The Greek physician, it has been said, wanted all successes and no failures. I suspect that such judgments are incorrect. Half of the number of patients reported on in Hippocrates' *Epidemics* (14 cases) died. The author not only "took his chances" but did not hesitate to report on the results.

Greek culture, and hence Greek medicine, was, so to say, tough-minded and realistic. Where Nature would not, or could not, how should the physician prevail? Also the Greeks had an attitude toward death quite different from our own. Plato speaks contemptuously of the man who though worn out by age or illness still would cling to life. Socrates, condemned to death, would not accept the advice of his friends to escape from prison and thus prolong his days among the living. It was, so he thought and so he acted, more fitting to accept Athens' judgment and to die.

Having shown, I hope, that Greek medicine was influenced by Greek culture, which was predominantly agrarian, I can now sketch its decline when the culture changed radically. For this I jump from the time of Hippocrates to the 16th century. The intervening period could also serve my purpose, for it embraced a series of cultural changes—the emergent dominance of Rome, the advent of Christianity, the Islamic conquests, etc.—which were reflected in the medicine of the period. Basically, however, Hippocratic medicine survived throughout the full stretch of time because the cultural changes were not truly radical. All the varying cultural orientations remained agricultural. The 16th century, however, witnessed the advent of the modern age with its commerce, mechanized industry, and analytical science, with its enormous increase in population and city dwelling. To this I would add the Reformation, with the emergence of what has been termed the Protestant Ethic. The cultural and technological revolution then begun brought with it a new order of morbidity, appropriately named by Major Greenwood, the crowd diseases

(3). Medicine in the Hippocratic tradition had little experience of these. The plague which broke out in Athens in 435 B.C. was attributable to the crowding of the Athenians into their capital to avoid the Lacadaemonians; and the crowd diseases of antiquity were only occasional results of crises, principally wars. Consequently, when those epidemic and endemic diseases "arose" from the conditions of life created by the new commercial and industrial civilization with its new ethos and new cultural characteristics, some change from Hippocratic ideas was needed. The task of medicine was no longer to mediate between errant Man and benevolent, beneficient Nature. Physical Nature itself had been assaulted, rough handled, dislodged from its appointed ways. At no time before in his long history had Man experienced so radical and so grievous a change in his many factored ecology—physical, functional, mental and moral!—and all in so short a time. Medicine was now called on to deal *not* with the man who transgressed Nature's ways, but rather with the noxious, morbifacient conditions and agents, products of new ways of life, which beset Man everywhere and at all times.

In the 16th century the denigration of Hippocratic medicine was signaled in the public burning of the books of Galen and Avicenna. It really matters little if the action ascribed to Paracelsus is fact or fancy. Hippocratic medicine had before this fallen into disrepute and disuse. New schools arose, sporting odd names, such as iatro-chemists and iatrophysicists. Common to these new schools of medical thought were the concepts of specific causative agents, including the *contagium vivum,* and specific curative agents. These concepts are still dominant in medicine.

Neither the epochal work of F. G. Hopkins nor that of Freud has made a dent in the persuasions or thinking patterns of the Specifist Aetiologic School. We still think in terms of specific causes and of specific cures and, what is more, we earnestly believe we have attained them.

But whether we have or not, this much appears certain; the cultural changes concomitant with the development of modern science and of modern economic and technological existence have had a profound influence on medicine. They have altered our ideas on the etiology of disease, on the role of the physician, and also on the place of death in human existence.

So far, then, I have cited medical history to support the thesis that medicine is *not* an exact science: It is not universally valid, nor is it independent of time, place and occasion. I have cited medical history to demonstrate that medicine is a discipline which, though it utilizes the exact sciences, is shaped and directed by cultural forces.

If this is true, it is important at several levels. In the first place, the history of medicine should no longer be formulated and presented as that of a science which was initially gross and corrupt but has been consistently refined and made more exact. It should be treated instead in terms of its cultural concomitants. Today, a great many people and institutions—politicians, government agencies, labor unions, welfare organizations, and so on—are affected by prevailing versions of medical history. Unconsciously they absorb the prevailing doctrinal generalizations. They suppose that diseases can be, have been, and will be *conquered*. Research, which is generally pictured in terms of complex laboratory operations, is the "royal road to the conquest of disease." Research is costly; but the more research is done, the sooner disease will be conquered.

Health is thought to depend on medical care, rendered by the physician. Hence, the more medical care is available to people, the better will be their health. And so on.

Such generalizations are not totally erroneous—only *ultimately* so. What is corect in them overlays and obscures what is grievously wrong; and a partial truth is frequently worse than a total error.

The advent of the modern socioeconomic-technological culture brought with it a new order of morbidities—the crowd diseases. But it did not eliminate the older ones, with which the Hippocratic physician was best acquainted. Nature did not abrogate its sovereignty. It was only that the crowd diseases preempted priority. The underlying dyscrasia was overlaid by the specific mortal morbidity.

I do not know that it could have been otherwise. But what *is* clear is that the crowd diseases, at least in the Western world, have now been brought largely under control. Consequently, more and more of our attention is claimed, once again, by the disorders of "faulty existence," the disorders that "do not kill" but make living "a trial," the functional, chronic, degenerative disorders. And the new challenge is, how are these to be dealt with?

The trend appears to be towards treating them along specifist lines. For the specific disorder diagnosed, a *specific* remedy, preferably pharmacological in nature, should be prescribed! The ideas and practice developed and applied in the control of the crowd diseases are now being extended and applied to the treatment of the predominantly functional disorders. A medical orientation developed in one cultural setting is being projected uncritically upon the medical problems of a radically different setting. I submit, were we to appreciate the interdependence of culture and medicine, were we to see the history of medicine in these relationships, we would be spared the incongruities we witness, experience and suffer today.

One final observation, this one touching on a matter as weighty as any dealt with thus far: What is to be the effect of the extension of Western medical theory and practice to the so-called underdeveloped countries? These countries have each their own historical indigenous medical systems. Are these to be discredited and discarded? Is Western medicine to be vaunted as science, and the indigenous systems branded as archaic, superstitious, ignorant? Must these countries, these peoples, inevitably repeat our blunders?

REFERENCES

1. Polanyi, M. *Science,* 1957, 125, 480-484.
2. *Ibid.,* p. 418.
3. Greenwood, M. *Epidemics and Crowd Diseases.* London: Williams & Norgate, 1935.

2

The Pathogenicity of Progress

Two considerations are here involved, pathogenicity and progress. What is meant by pathogenic is clear enough. It refers to a quality that engenders a disturbance in the normal, which ultimately results in disease. But progress is a nebulous and relative term. We speak, for example, of "social progress" and likewise of the "progress" of a disease process leading to death. The sense in which I intend the term progress is fairly specific, referring in the main to social and economic advance. I premise therein those technological developments which in a Spencerian sense effect a social passage from the simple to the complex, and from the homogeneous to the heterogeneous. Implied in such change is a concomitant radical ecological change, and the pathogenicity of progress specifically derives from this change.

There are many historical instances that can be cited to illustrate this postulation. Some of the more recent ones are perhaps the more easy to appreciate. Thus, the development of the antibiotics represents a significant technological advance. By means of these antibacterial agents, the death of many individuals has been and is deferred. The immediate results are an increase in total population, and a change in the age distribution of that population, with a marked increment in the older age segment. This assuredly is progress. It is also 'pathogenic.' It is *progress* when, by means of the antibiotic or other chemotherapeutic agent, the parturient mother is spared from heretofore generally fatal effects of a septicemia, or the old man is saved from the mortal issue of a serious pneumonia. It is *pathogenic* when, as in the countries of limited economic and agricultural competences and resources, widespread and grievous malnutrition follows reduction of the infant death-rate (1).

The pathogenicity of progress may be social as well as biological. An appreciable proportion of new admissions to State mental hospitals are of so-called seniles. *When* one becomes senile and by what criteria one is to be adjudged so are to a large extent moot issues. Seemingly, it should be easy to determine the "competence" of a person. But, in effect, very much depends on the setting in which competence is tested. The country road is one setting and the New York subway system quite another. The man who is at home in the one can easily become disoriented in the other. Senility, therefore, may be, and frequently is, the diagnostic product of an equation in which endowment is the numerator and exacting circumstances the denominator. Exacting circumstances are, not infrequently, a collateral of progress.

Technologic unemployment is another instance of "pathology resulting from progress." Technological unemployment, initially socioeconomic in character, cannot long remain free of biological consequences, untoward in nature.

Many other examples can be cited. Leisure—that is, free time to be utilized at will—is a gain which man has sought since he was, for his sins, driven out of the Garden of Eden and condemned to earn his bread by the sweat of his brow. This curse, at least for a great number of the Western pepole, has been lifted. The work week which a century ago was of seventy-two hours duration has now been reduced by nearly half (2). Free time has been increased accordingly. But now, unstructured leisure has become a problem unique in the history of mankind, and one that is not without serious sociobiological consequences. Peoples' efforts to escape the boredom of unstructured leisure yield a spectacular array of disorders.

The crowning example perhaps is this: Thanks to what is termed "medical progress," Man now threatens to swamp the earth with his own kind—so that the world's population which currently is counted as over four billion will, "unless something appallingly bad or miraculously good should happen in the interval," be six billion by the year 2000 (3).

The development of ataraxic drugs is, without doubt, a boon to the psychiatrically sick and to the psychiatric hospitals. Yet the return to the community of so many sick who had been, some of them, confined in institutions for years and decades is not without disadvantages. Not every family is capable of accepting and reintegrating what, in effect, is a resurrected member. Nor is the larger community always ready to reabsorb the returned individual.

These examples should suffice to show what is intended by the "pathogenicity of progress," and perchance also to validate the tie between the one and the other. I must, however, hasten to make clear that the foregoing is not intended as an argument to "Stop Progress." Nor is it a plea for what is termed social Darwinism. Confessedly, I do not know whether it would be preferable to die of diarrhea at the age of nine months or of kwashiorkor at the age of six years. I do not even know how right the ancient sage was who opined that only that man is fortunate who was never born. In a word, no moral, social or even esthetic conclusion is intended or is to be drawn from the postulation on the pathogenicity of progress.

But there *is* an historic relevance to all this, for the pathogenicity of progress has a bearing on the comprehension of medical historical happenings, and hence also on historiography. For, where one encounters a nodal point in general history—marked by a "spurt of progress," of the nature previously defined—one may also expect to find some order of new, novel, and/or much intensified pathology. Conversely, one needs to look for some "episode of marked progress," one that radically affects and changes the given ecology, to help account for the appearance of new and intensified pathologies. (Total explanations are outside the realm of the possible.)

Need I affirm the obvious, that pathogenicity is not solely associated with progress, but may also be a concomitant of *regression*—and even of *static immobility?* The latter two associations are well appreciated, but that with 'progress' far less.

To illustrate in more detail the pathogenicity of progress, let us take the great epidemics of the Middle Ages. Several major factors can be recognized in their causation, and each was a nodal point on the scale of progress. These were: the extensive deforestation of Europe to gain more arable land; a considerable increase in population; the revival, growth and development of large cities; and the development of commerce and industry.

First in this series was the agricultural revolution that occurred between the 11th and the middle of the 14th centuries. During this period, inspired and guided by the religious Orders, notably the Cistercians, vast stretches of land were cleared of forest, brush and scrub. "An immense programme was . . . quietly carried out for the conquest of the littorals, river valleys and marshes, and for the clearance of heaths and forests" (4). Agriculture itself was improved. The soil was manured with both vegetable and animal matter, and was improved by the addition of complementary soil conditioners such as chalk, marl, ashes, turf and calcerous sand (5). The iron ploughshare, drawn by powerful teams of oxen or horses, was employed extensively, and the earth was thus ploughed more deeply, often seven or eight times on end.

Food production increased everywhere. And everywhere population increased. The West, which had been depopulated by the "barbarian invasions," was peopled again with extraordinary rapidity in the space of three hundred years (6). At the beginning of the 14th century, Western Europe contained together some 60 million souls—twice as many as before the 5th century (7). Unhappily, much of this increased crop of humans became surplus population. The prevailing feudal economy could not absorb them.

> The younger sons of a man, overburdened with children, were often forced to leave their father in order to enable him to make payments to the Lord. Thenceforth, they swelled the crowd of vagabonds, who roamed through the country, going from abbey to abbey taking their share of alms reserved for the poor, hiring themselves out to the peasants at harvest time or at vintage, and enlisting as mercenaries in the feudal troops in times of war (8).

Many, however, turned to the cities. "The increase of population," Pirenne wrote, "naturally favoured industrial concentration. Numbers of the poor poured into the towns [where] trade grew proportionately with the development of commerce [and] guaranteed them their daily bread" (9).

As was to be expected, their condition was pitiable. Unorganized and competing with one another for the work available, they were paid a miserable wage.

Little wonder, then, that in the 14th century Europe was racked by catastrophes and social disturbances. The earliest and most devastating famine occurred between 1315 and 1317. But on the score of famine and death, it is to be held in mind that they were the results as much of the more numerous mouths to be fed as of the lesser quantities of food available.

In 1348 the Black Death appeared in Europe, and estimates suggest that more than a quarter of the population perished from it. The 14th century, in effect, experienced the ravages of many epidemic diseases, including leprosy, typhus, dysentery and smallpox. In these epidemics we may perceive the beginnings of what Major Greenwood so aptly termed the *crowd diseases* (10)—diseases which initially found a fertile soil in the walled towns of feudal Europe with their cramped and unwholesome manner of life, inhabited spots of ground choked with the waste matter of generations (11).

Wars, famines, epidemics, civil strife, revolts by peasants and by workers, religious schisms, heresies and factions mark the 14th century as one of grievous turmoil and disorder. Yet the preceding two hundred and fifty years are celebrated as the Golden period of the Middle Ages, a period that saw great progress. During this period commercial activity was revived and industrial production increased. Town life was animated and movable wealth, in contrast to fixed land, increased. A new order of the working class, grouped in the towns, emerged to gain both power and liberty. Through their craft organizations and their sworn corporations they gained recognition for the social value of their labor, and "raised themselves to a level of material and moral existence unknown to their forebears" (12). Yet the century following—the 14th—was one of widespread and profound misery. Here, too, progress proved pathogenic.

It seems odd that historians have paid so little attention to the relation between progress and its pathological consequences. I am aware of but one modern thinker who has studied these matters in depth. Ortega y Gasset has explored them in *Man and Crisis* (13), though his concerns are chiefly with the moral and the ethical. Yet perhaps it is, after all, not so strange that the pathogenicity of progress has been so little recognized. Science discarded its ecological orientation more than three hundred years ago. It cannot, therefore, easily appreciate that *progress,* which in its true and primary order (and as we have defined it) is always innovational—not merely elaborative, always has a disruptive effect on the ecosystem (14). The pathogenic effects derive from this disruption.

But if some disruption is inevitable, its degree and kind are not. In reconstructing the social and economic edifice, it is not inescapably necessary that it be torn down about the heads of its occupants and that they be buried in the debris. That this happens more often than not should seriously interest historians, sociologists, and statesmen.

REFERENCES

1. For a succinct summary of the issues, see: Lucas, F. L., *The Greatest Problem.* New York: Macmillan, 1961, p. 299; and *The Human Sum,* C. H. Rolph, Ed. New York: Macmillan, 1957.
2. Dewhurst, J. F., et al. *American Needs and Resources.* New York: Twentieth Century Fund, 1947, p. 23.
3. Woytinsky, W. S. & E. S. *World Population and Production.* New York: Twentieth Century Fund, 1953, p. 367.
4. Boissonnade, P. *Life and Work in Medieval Europe.* London: Routledge, 1927, p. 227.

5. *Ibid.*, p. 234.
6. *Ibid.*, p. 237.
7. *Ibid.*, p. 238.
8. Pirenne, H. *Economic and Social History of Medieval Europe.* New York: Harcourt Brace, 1936, p. 45.
9. Pirenne, H. *Medieval Cities.* New York: Doubleday, 1925, p. 110.
10. Greenwood, M. *Epidemics and Crowd Diseases.* London: William & Norgate, 1935.
11. Creighton, C. *History of Epidemics in Britain,* 2 vols. Cambridge University Press, 1891, vol. 1, p. 175.
12. Boissonnade, P. *op. cit.*, p. 333.
13. Ortega y Gasset, J. *Man and Crisis.* New York: Norton, 1958.
14. Sauer, C. O. The agency of man on the earth. In: *Man's Role in Changing the Face of the Earth,* W. L. Thomas, Jr., Ed. University of Chicago Press, 1956, p. 68.

3

Technology, Culture and Disease

Mankind's first and most significant technological innovation was the making of fire. That, according to Linton, took place some thirty thousand years ago (1). Man *used* fire for at least a quarter million years. But he has *made* fire only during the last thirty thousand years (2). This great technological innovation is embodied in the myth of Prometheus, who stole fire from Zeus and gave it to Man. Because of that transgression, Zeus cruelly punished him. This myth is propounded in the Theogony of Hesiod and magnificently elaborated in the Promethean plays of Aeschylus. But whereas Hesiod saw Prometheus only as the Evil One, who was properly punished, Aeschylus, with that mighty imaginative power which we cannot sufficiently admire and honor, built up his act into an imperishable symbol of humanity.

"Prometheus he made the Bringer of Light to suffering mankind. The divine power of fire was for him the concrete image of civilization. And Prometheus was the civilizing genius who explores the whole world, who makes it subservient to his will by organizing its forces, who reveals its treasures and establishes on a firm basis the groping, insecure life of man" (3).

Aeschylus was not a scientist, but a poet-dramatist steeped in the wisdom of cosmic harmony. He well understood, and superbly expounded the essence of the Promethean tragedy. "Aeschylus," writes Werner Jaeger, "did not conceive that the Titan's sin was merely an offense against the property of the gods, consisting in the theft of their fire, but rather (in accordance with the spiritual and symbolic significance which he imparted to it) that it was connected with some deep tragic imperfection in the benefit he had done to mankind by his wonderful gift" (4).

This tragic imperfection lay in Prometheus' failure to grasp what

Anaximander, the Ionian philosopher, so clearly affirmed, namely, that the ecologic concordance may not be tampered with save at the cost of "penalty and compensation." "Things," Anaximander stated, "must pay one another the penalty and compensation for their injustices according to the ordinance of time" (5). The fault of Prometheus, then, lay in that he did not anticipate the penalties and compensations that mankind would be required to bear and to render—because he had breached the accord set up by Zeus.

In the classical period the Greeks substituted for the "accord set by Zeus" the more rational concept of *physis*—translated in English as Nature. The Ionian term *physis,* however, means something more than its nominal equivalent in English. Nature, in its English version, usually comprehends the sum total or aggregate of natural things. To the Ionians, physis-nature always meant *that something* inhering in things which makes them behave as they do (6). Such to the Greeks was its essential meaning, but its logical extension also embraced the concepts of Nature as a real thing, as a unity, and postulated the existence of substance, of matter, in which behavior becomes manifest.*

It is in this light that the argument expounded in the Hippocratic book *On the Nature of Man* can best be understood. Indeed, it is in this light that the totality of Hippocratic-Galenic medicine is to be understood. Hippocratic-Galenic medicine is ecological in viewpoint and persuasion, ecology being the science of the relation of things. It embodies the archaic "accord set up by Zeus," the Anaximandrian "commerce and contract between things" and the *physis* of classical Greece and of Hippocratic medicine.

"There had always been doctors," writes Werner Jaeger, "but the craft of healing in Greece had not developed into a methodological science sure of its aim until it felt the influence of Ionian natural philosophy" (7).

Medicine itself depended on the concept of the great *physis,* the Nature of the Universe—the idea developed by Ionian philosophy. "The introduction of the treatise *On Airs, Waters and Places* is a splendid expression of the way in which Hippocratean medical thought depends on the philosophical view of nature as a whole" (8). Hippocratic-Galenic medicine survived the disintegration of the Greco-Roman world and pre-

* They took their myths but not always their lessons in earnest. The Greek demos had as little regard for the accord set up by Zeus or for the teachings of Anaximander as does the present-day apartment house janitor whose incinerator belches its smoke and fumes into the atmosphere. The pernicious Greek goat helped to denude the Attican plains and mountains.

vailed, though corrupted, throughout the Mediterranean lands, Europe, and the Arabic realms.

With the advent of the Renaissance, however, Hippocratic medicine was challenged and then rejected, as was the Ionian philosophy of *physis.* Derivatively, the validity of the ecologic concept was also rejected.

For the Renaissance thinkers, the natural world was not, as it was for the Greek, an organism governed by an indwelling intelligence. It was, rather, a machine in the literal and proper sense of the word, an arrangement of bodily parts designed, put together and set going for a definite purpose by an intelligent mind outside itself. In the early stages of the Renaissance, the intelligence outside of Nature was identified with God of Judeo-Christianity, the divine creator and ruler of Nature. Historically it was but a brief step from this to dismissal of the celestial pilot, an action tersely expressed in a remark by Laplace. When Napoleon asked him how he had managed to write a book on the Creation without mentioning the Creator, he replied: "Je n'avais pas besoin de cette hypothèse-là." God was not dead, he was merely replaced by the modern scientist, in whose wake followed the modern technologist.*

We have come a long way from the time thirty thousand or more years ago when Prometheus, the first major technological innovator, stole fire from the gods. In the interval there were many other innovational technologists, not the least among them the brother of Prometheus, Epimetheus, who is credited with having invented marriage and the family (9).**

The mastery of fire-making made possible numerous other technologies, the smelting of metals, the baking of pottery, the clearing of forest lands, and—as significant as any—cooking. It can indeed be said that all the known technological innovations derive from the original one—making fire.

It is, of course, not possible here to review even the major advances. But it should be noted that the conjunction of innovation and human misery has been commented on since myths were forged and history was written. Thus the myth of a Golden Age is almost universal. Hesiod, in *Works and Days,* tells of five generations of men, the first a golden race

* In the strict sense of the terms "scientist" and "technologist," the relationship between the two is not quite correctly stated above. In many instances the skillful draftsman, the technologist, initiated the innovation, the scientist coming after to explain and to reduce to scientific terms and also to perfect what the craftsman-technologist had begun and accomplished.

** It is amusing to read Hesiod's comments on this significant technological advance. He finds it difficult to decide where the advantages lie, in bachelorhood or marriage.

of mortal men who lived like gods without sorrow of heart and free from toil and grief; of the last, the fifth, Hesiod's own generation, he bewails, "Would that I were not among the men of the fifth generation, but either had died before or been born afterwards" (10). But though bewailed and lamented, no generation of men until our own had the wisdom or summoned up the courage to face the inevitable challenge of innovation, that of ecological and cultural disorientation with its attendant miseries.

Though here concerned with technological innovation, we need bear in mind that innovations occur in other realms as well, in the cultural, aesthetic, ideational, to name but several. The innovations embodied in the concepts of evolution and the Freudian unconscious also proved very upsetting. They painfully upset traditional beliefs and modes of thought. The Spanish philosopher, Ortega y Gasset, has dealt with this order of innovation, distinct and apart from technology, in his excellent work *Man and Crisis* (11).

Until the 16th century, innovation was frequently resisted, often lamented, and inevitably suffered. Then, with the advent of modern science, innovation became a prime achievement to be sought and prized. It was henceforth looked upon as the sovereign means and way of Progress, and Progress was enshrined as the great human ideal. Progress had no upper price limit; whatever it cost, it was a bargain.

To such a persuasion ecology was an alien and repugnant concept. It was romantic, and reactionary! Admittedly, innovation, summed up as progress, brought with it much human misery and suffering. But that was inescapable. "At the heart of the Industrial Revolution of the 18th century (when modern technology had passed the toddler's stage) there was an almost miraculous improvement in the tools of productions, which was accompanied by a catastrophic dislocation of the lives of the common people" (12). "The laboring people had been crowded together in new places of desolation . . . the country folk had been dehumanized into slum dwellers; the family was on the road to perdition; and large parts of the country were rapidly disappearing under the slack and scrap heaps vomited forth from the 'Satanic mills'" (13). And all of this seemed inevitable; indeed, by some it was looked upon as good. Jeremiah Bentham believed that poverty was part of plenty. "In the highest stage of social prosperity," he wrote, "the great mass of citizens will most probably possess no other resources than their daily labor, and consequently will always be near to indigence" (14).*

* In 1704 Daniel Defoe published a pamphlet titled *Alms No Charity and Employing the Poor a Grievance to the Nation.*

Among the 18th century thinkers it was generally agreed that pauperism and progress were inseparable. Only Robert Owen, forerunner of Social Darwinism, disassociated himself from this philosophy.

How had the social conscience become so blunted? Two observations may be ventured, one pointing to the prevailing religious mood, the other to the prevailing image of Nature. The religious mood, primarily Protestant in derivation, looked to God not only as the Creator and prime mover of the universe, but also as the sovereign regulator of Man's affairs on earth. If there be poor among us, it is by God's will, as it is also His wish that the rich and the favored should be charitable to the poor. The religious mood is well mirrored in a paper written by the distinguished churchman William Paley titled *Reasons for Contentment Addressed to the Labouring Part of the British Public.* In this work Paley argues, "Some of the necessities which poverty (if the condition of the labouring part of mankind must be so called) imposes, are not hardships but pleasures. Frugality itself is a pleasure. It is an exercise of attention and contrivance, which whenever it is successful, produces satisfaction. The very care and forecast that are necessary to keep expenses and earnings upon a level form, when not embarrassed by too great difficulties, are an agreeable engagement of the thoughts. This is lost amidst abundance" (15).

The prevailing image of Nature was, as already noted, that of a complex machine, geared and regulated in its various parts by laws which were innate to it. There were economic laws, social laws, laws of political life, laws of the market, of labor, of capital and so forth. These were inexorable and inviolable laws, not to be tampered with save at great peril. Hence the injunction Laissez-faire, laissez-aller. This version of Nature with its inexorable laws was greatly reinforced during the 19th century by the theories of organic evolution as propounded by Charles Darwin and of social evolution as advanced by Herbert Spencer. Evolution was accepted as a regulatory force operating within Nature to assure the selection, the survival and the multiplication of the fittest! The twain, God and Nature, were thus accepted as "knowing best" and it was impious and irrational for man to interfere with the ways of either.

In the concluding chapter of his learned and thoughtful book *What is History?*, Edward Carr writes, "in the 17th and 18th centuries man had already become fully conscious of the world around him and its laws. They were no longer the mysterious decrees of an inscrutable providence, but laws accessible to reason. But they were laws to which Man was subject, and not laws of his own making. In the next stage man was to become fully conscious of his power over his environment and over himself and of his right to make the laws under which he would live" (16). This, Professor Carr regards as the major feature of the 20th century revolution—that by the application of rational processes, Man will be enabled to improve the management of his social, economic and political affairs (17). Of this there can be no doubt, but it decisively depends on the conceptual framework within which Man will exercise the rational processes. If it is not within the ecological, the result will at best be failure and at worst be disaster.

Professor Carr leaves one uneasy on this score. He celebrates the abandonment of faith in and submission to the so-called objective laws of social, political, economic life. He appears, however, to firmly believe that by taking thought (which does not include the ecological) Man can become sovereign master of himself and the universe. This is a dangerous belief, unwarranted and unsupported in historic experience. It is to this hazard that I believe Professor Eric Weil directed the following comments: "Science and its offspring, technology, have come to stay, and we shall have to live with them. The question is, first, how we are to do so without producing more and more split personalities, particularly among the best educated and most serious people, and, second, how we are to prevent those drunk with this new power from exercising in our name the acquired mastery over Nature and history in order to dominate us for domination's sake" (18). In the same issue of *Daedalus,* Oscar Handlin wrote, "The people who are simultaneously delighted with additional years of life expectancy and terrified by the bomb are in no position to strike the balance of their gains and losses in happiness. In their confusion, they wonder whether the price of the gadgets which delight may not be servitude to the remote and alien few who control the mystery" (19).

These two quotations, to which many others could be added, show that there is a keen, widespread and anxious awareness that our new technology confronts society with challenge and menace. It is encouraging and somewhat reassuring that there is this awareness. No previous age facing a truly radical technological innovation attained a similar awareness of challenge and menace. The question now to be asked is, what are we to do with this awareness? Here we must confine our query to medicine; and the question I shall consider is what disabilities are likely to result from the ecological upset which the new technologies will unquestionably cause in our immediate world and everyday living. For the challenge to medicine today is not only to adapt its practice to the age of computers, electronic diagnostic tools, synthetic chemotherapeutic agents, the marvels of tissue and organ transplantation, the webs of bureaucracy and government medicine, and the rest, but also to make ready to meet the miseries and sicknesses that perforce will come in the wake of the new technology.

In the earlier technological revolutions it was the earth itself, its forests and animal inhabitants, that bore the brunt. Mankind was not exempt, but in the main Man thrived; though once a rare mammal, he became one of the most numerous and widespread among them. It is believed that "the entire population of the earth after men had been wandering and increasing for a quarter of a million of years probably did not number as many persons as in the city of New York today" (21).

In the more recent technological revolutions, those of modern industrialism, embracing the development and use of water power, machines, the steam engine, the internal combustion engine, electric power and fractional electric motors, mankind was more intimately involved and more deeply affected. Perhaps the most significant of the ecological changes Man experienced was urbanization, the withdrawal of men from the country and their herding into numerous towns and cities. Beyond that for many hundreds of thousands there came a herding, during daytime, into shops and factories, and at night into tenements. "The routine of the farmer," wrote Oscar Hendlin, "had been coordinate with the forces of the visible world around him, or at least it seems so. The alterations of the seasons told him when to plant and when to reap; the rising and the setting sun told him when to begin his labors and when to rest. The machine disregarded all such considerations and operated at its own pace, winter and summer, day and night. The new regime detached work from the other aspects of life" (22). And it detached Man from the natural forces that should regulate his life. The result, in the piercing phrase of Karl Polanyi, was "a society which had forgotten the shape of man" (21).

The technologies of the industrial revolution did indeed affect "the shape of man." Those of the confronting revolution threaten to change Man's ethos. Urbanization brought with it the crowd diseases. What order of new diseases will the newer technologies bring with them? For ever and above all the great promises of automation, cybernation, data processing, and a fully computerized existence, there stands this stark, fearful menace, that the values which man has lived by and prized, those of diligent work, of thrift, of individual initiative, of charity, of mutual aid, of intimate shared responsibilities within the family and beyond in the community—all these and others beside will be rendered nugatory. Already a number of them have lost their pertinence to present-day life, and there is little prospect that they will ever be redeemed. It may be thought that this is a moral challenge and hence should be left to the moral leaders to be dealt with. It will be their charge, too, but moral issues are not without their medical components. Indeed, as in the case of alcoholism, the venereal diseases, obesity, and other diseases, numerous issues acquire moral significance precisely because they are medically urgent. But it may be further asked, how can a vanishing ethos prove pathogenic? Here I can do no better than to quote Ortega y Gasset: "An historical crisis occurs when . . . the system of convictions belonging to a previous generation gives way to a vital state in which man remains without these convictions, and therefore without a world." And further: "Crisis man has been left without a world, handed over to the chaos of pure circumstances, in a lamentable state of disorganization. On feeling himself lost, man may respond with skeptical frigidity, with anguish, or with desperation; and he will do many things, which though apparently heroic, do not in fact proceed from any real heroism but are deeds done in desperation. Or he will have a sense of fury, of madness, and appetite for vengeance, because of the emptiness of his life; these will drive him to enjoy brutally, cynically, whatever comes his way—flesh, luxury, power. Life takes on a bitter flavor" (11). It is thus that a vanishing ethos becomes pathogenic.

Zbigniew Brzezinski of Columbia University published in 1966 a most luminous article titled "Tomorrow's Agenda" (23). His thesis is proximate to my own and I cite him freely. His premise is that in the second half of the 20th century the developed nations, given new scientific and social developments, will face a real threat to the continued existence of Man as a spontaneous, instinctive, rather autonomous and even somewhat mysterious being. A social revolution already in progress is likely to be shaped by the widespread adoption of automation and cybernation for social and economic reasons. Men's environment and Man himself will more and more be subject to purposive control and manipulation. Our society will be fundamentally transformed. Our concepts of work and leisure will most likely undergo a basic reversal, leisure becoming a burden and creative work a privilege of the gifted few. The relationship between employment and way of life will be revised. Retirement and unemployment, the basic social functions of trade unions and of government welfare operations, will most likely undergo radical revision. The relationship between earning and consumption will be blurred, with the prospects of arbitrary standards to assure a minimum level of consumption. Within such changes, how is the integrity and freedom of Man as an individual to be preserved? Given the trends in medical sciences, as a physical being Man will become more malleable, and as a personality, subject increasingly to external manipulations. The more Man is thus manipulated and programmed, the increasingly more denatured he is likely to become. The extended result is likely to be personal and political alienation and a pervasive sense of seemingly purposeless lives.

All of these are likely eventualities. They are concomitants of the new technologies, and carry with them the prospects of a host of new medical problems. Medicine must seek to anticipate them, to meet them, and to deal with them effectively. Medicine must also be prepared to intelligently counsel government and other social groups and organizations. This, among other things, calls for a critical look at present-day medical education, to assess whether and how we can in time educate and train physicians competent to meet the emergent medical needs of the new society; whether, in the large sense, we can effect, and in the world of our professional concern see to it, that the penalties and compensations which things owe to one another in the changed ecology are paid out in time and in good coin.

REFERENCES

1. Linton, R. & Linton, A. *Man's Way From Cave to Skyscraper.* New York: Harper, 1947, p. 26.
2. Stewart, O. C. Fire as the first great force employed by Man. In: *Man's Role in Changing the Face of the Earth,* W. L. Thomas, Jr., Ed. University of Chicago Press, 1956, p. 117.
3. Jaeger, W. *Paideia: The Ideals of Greek Culture.* New York: Oxford University Press, 1945, vol. 1, p. 262.
4. *Ibid.,* p. 264.
5. *Ibid.,* p. 160.
6. Collingwood, R. G. *The Idea of Nature.* New York: Oxford University Press, 1945, p. 44.
7. Jaeger, W. *op. cit.,* Vol. III, p. 5.
8. Jaeger, W. *op. cit.,* Vol. III, p. 6.
9. Hesiod, *Theogony.* 600-613.
10. Hesiod. *Works and Days.* 110-115, 174-180.
11. Ortega y Gasset, J. *Man and Crisis.* New York: Norton, 1958, p. 86-88.
12. Polanyi, K. *Origins of Our Time.* London: Gollancz, 1945, p. 41.
13. *Ibid.,* p. 47.
14. Bentham, J. *Principles of Civil Code,* p. 314, (cited by Polanyi, *op. cit.,* p. 121).
15. Cited by Hammond, J. L. & Hammond, B. *The Town Labourer (1760-1832).* New York: Longmans, 1920, p. 233.
16. Carr, E. H. *What is History?* New York: Knopf, 1965, p. 180.
17. *Ibid.,* p. 190.

18. WEIL, E. Science in modern culture, or the meaning of meaninglessness. *Daedalus,* Winter 1965, p. 186.
19. HANDLIN, O. Science and technology in popular culture. *Daedalus,* Winter 1965, p. 170.
20. LINTON, R. & LINTON, A. *op. cit.,* p. 14.
p. 14.
21. POLANYI, K. *op. cit.,* p. 169.
22. HANDLIN, O. Man and magic: First encounters with the machine. *The American Scholar,* Summer 1964, p. 410.
23. BRZEZINSKI, Z. Tomorrow's agenda. *Foreign Affairs Quarterly Review,* July 1966.

4

Manipulator, Scientist, Wastrel

The myth of Prometheus magnificently propounds the tragic complex of *Homo sapiens* and *Homo faber,* of Man who lives both within and without the "accord set up by Zeus." For Man's unresolved problem, now as in the mythic days of Prometheus, is how to alter the world about him to suit his needs and wishes, thereby inescapably altering the ecology, and yet not suffer such dire penalties and retributive compensations as will undo both him and his world.

From his very beginning Man was a manipulator of his environment, in ways and degrees so much greater than those of any other living creature that he was set apart from all the rest. He was also a creature uniquely curious about everything. In that sense, since he was not merely curious but sought to understand, he was a scientist from the start. But he had no thought of becoming master of his world. He lived within Nature and not, so to say, outside it.

For changing his environment, fire was one of his earliest tools. He has used it for at least a quarter of a million years (1), and it served him in many different ways. He set fire to jungles and thick woods to open them up so that hunting would be better and safer. He set fire to rouse and drive game, to improve pasture, to increase berry crops, and as a means of war.

But the most important use of fire was to increased Man's food supply. It greatly extended the kinds of vegetable foods he could eat and digest. Meats can be eaten uncooked, and so can some wild fruits, nuts and berries. But most root vegetables, tubers, and grains, the staples of the vegetable crop, cannot be consumed raw. As Linton phrased it, "Bread is man's staff of life but there can be not bread without fire" (2).

Fire and increased food yielded a marked increase in population, Man's early boon and threatening bane.

Though early Man burned extensive areas, over and over again, his activities are thought to have had little if any effect on the geographic environment. Nor was the potential fertility of the soil, or, in general, Man's ecology, radically changed during the period of classical antiquity, i.e. from 1100 B.C. to the 6th cenutry A.D. What did change at that time were Man's social patterns, his intellectual and political orientations, and his technological competences, the latter having grown immensely.

One of the most radical ecological changes took place during the early part of the present millenium, and it derived from technological improvements in agriculture. These, in turn, increased the population. For food production and population are interdependent. An increase in food production favors an increase in population. The latter then becomes a pressure source for greater food production, and the continuing interreaction causes a spiraling of both.

At the beginning of the Christian era, the population of the Roman Empire, including slaves, was approximately 55 million, of whom 23 million inhabited Europe and the rest Africa (14.5 million) and Asia (17.5 million). Six hundred years later, because of the disintegration of the Roman Empire, the ensuing wars, famines and plagues, Europe's population had declined to below 20 million. Conditions were even worse during the next four hundred years. But at some point during this dismal period a reaction set in in the form of "agrarian colonization." Men began to extend the arable lands. "For," as Bennett wrote, "to a family burdened with more children than their shares in the common fields would warrant . . . assart land (that is, land free to be cleared and used) was a godsend. Here they could utilise their spare labour, and produce something to help fill the many hungry mouths at home" (3).

Clearing the land meant cutting down trees and grubbing up roots—arduous and back-breaking labor. Yet it was done, consistently and effectively. The arable land was greatly extended, and Europe largely deforested.

In the time of Charlemagne (742-814 A.D.), forests spread their cloak over a great part of the soil of the West. Ireland, Wales, Cornwall, and the Scottish Highlands, which are today bare, were then covered with vast oak, birch, fir, and pine woods. A third of Flanders and the Netherlands, now so bare, were, before the 11th century, largely forest regions, joining on to the immense forests of the Ardennes and the Eifel. Germany and France were heavily forested. "From Argonne to the Alps and the Pyrenees, from the Ocean to the Juras, all was forest, interspersed with open plains which had been brought under cultivation" (4). Within these forests there were quantities of bears, boars, deer and stags, bisons, aurochs and beavers.

Forests and animals were ruthlessly sacrificed to gain more arable land to feed more hungry humans. Beginning about the year 1000, there began a period of land reclamation which was to continue, intensively, to the end of the 12th century, and with an abated intensity up to our own days. "At no period," wrote Boissonnade, "has the conquest of agricultural land been carried on with so much discipline and ardour" (5). Thousands of pioneers came to prepare the way for the work of plough and hoe by burning away brushwood, thickets, and parasitic vegetation, clearing forests with the axe, and uprooting trunks with the pick. As a result, the face of Europe changed. "Germany in particular was transformed. In its immense forests, through some of which an eleventh-century missionary could ride for five days on end in complete solitude, pioneers made clearings, . . . established great farms all along the side of the roads or on the edge of the woods" (6). In England the woods were attacked with such vigor that nothing was left of the ancient forest which once covered the soil of Britain, save a few rare remnants. In the Low Countries, France, Spain and Italy, the forest fell before the axe of the pioneer, and with this a pitiless war was waged against wild beasts.

The plough followed in the wake of axe and pick. "Side by side with the labor of hoe and spade, the use of the iron ploughshare allowed the earth to be plowed deeply, sometimes seven or eight times on end" (7). Improved ploughing and manuring of the land, along with superior cultivation of cereals and of vegetables, yielded better harvests and a larger food resource for both animals and humans. In consequence, by the end of the 13th century the population of the six states of the West contained together perhaps 60 million souls, twice as many as they had numbered before the 5th century (8). But the Middle Ages had frequent years of famine (9), and to the terrors of starvation were added those of great epidemics, as we saw in considering *The Pathogenicity of Progress* —epidemics arising partly because more and more people lived in towns which were overcrowded.

During the million or so years since his emergence and up to the advent of modern science, Man had acquired a great deal of scientific, technological, philosophical, and psychological lore. The distinctive feature of that scientific lore was that, in the main, it served to explain, to make understandable, to give an account of the world about, and of one's experience in it. The older science was not experimental, but rather observational and descriptive. It was also conjectural, or, as we say today, deductive. For the older generations of Man, the world itself was the laboratory, and existence the experiment. All this implied a basic acceptance of the world, and also of Nature, as that given whole within which all efforts to "better things" must perforce be confined. To paraphrase and sum up, the underlying conviction was that the world could be bettered, but not changed.

In the early part of the last millenium, this heretofore solid faith was breached by a beginning doubt. Precisely *when* is hard to say, and the reasons *why* even more so. Since history is commonly anchored to personages, we might cite the name of Roger Bacon, Franciscan monk, born about the year 1210. He was greatly ahead of his time, in that he was an advocate of the experimental method. He himself conducted some research in a number of problems, with, however, meager results. He "foresaw" many mechanical inventions, such as machine-driven ships, carriages, and flying boats. He toyed with a host of items such as burning glasses, gunpowder, the magnet, Greek fire, and artificial gold. Roger Bacon is, in a sense, an anomaly, rather than an innovator. His impact upon his contemporaries was negligible. But he did foreshadow the coming age of scientific inquiry, the age we call the Renaissance.

The effective heralds of that age were Copernicus (1473-1543), Telesio (1508-1588) and Giordano Bruno (1548-1600). These were the initiators of the persuasion that differed so radically from the one held by the ancients, namely, that the world moved in the "accord set up by Zeus." The world of nature, these innovators maintained, is not an organism guided by intelligence. The natural world, they argued, is a machine: a machine in the literal and proper sense of the word. "The Renaissance thinkers," wrote Collingwood, "like the Greeks, saw in the orderliness of the natural world an expression of intelligence: but for the Greeks this intelligence was nature's own intelligence, for the Renaissance thinkers it was the intelligence of something other than Nature: the divine creator and ruler of nature" (10).

The Greeks understood the meaning of ecology and they understood its dynamics. So, too, did the medieval thinkers. They viewed man as the lesser image of the greater universe, the microcosm of the macrocosm. But with the advent of modern science, this insight into the interrelationship of man with the rest of the world, both living and inanimate, was obscured. Science dazzled man's vision, and the tragedy of Prometheus was compounded a "thousand thousandfold."

Now Man spoke not of the "accord set up by Zeus," or of its equivalent, but of "mastering nature." "Men no longer studied macrocosm and microcosm as such," wrote Singer, "but they became physicists or physiologists, taking each of them a separated portion of the universe for special study" (11).

The high priest of this new devotion was Francis Bacon. His *Novum Organum* most clearly expounds the spirit of the new and dawning age of modern science. Therein he propounded his theory of science as the means to discovery and invention. But his was not an idle curiosity, nor a vain pursuit. Bacon was a very practical man and thinker. A science that is not practically useful was, in Bacon's eyes, worth nothing. By means of science, Bacon argued, it would be possible to establish the "dominion of man," the *regnum hominis,* over all things, so that the wants of Man's life might be satisfied, his pleasure multiplied, and his power increased. The dominion of Man over things, Bacon urged, is the highest and indeed the sole end of science (12).

No thought here, then, of ecology, no vision of the tribute things must pay to things, nor the awareness of the penalties to be paid according to the ordinance of time when injustices are inflicted.

Francis Bacon is one of the more famous names associated with the dawn of modern science, but he was not one of the founders of science. He was one of its early philosophers and advocates. "Bacon comprehended the altered physiognomy of his age; he sought for the ultimate causes of the change, and wished to make philosophy accord with it. For the new life and its impulses he wished to find a new corresponding logic" (13). He did, and it turned out to be the logic of man's dominance over all things.

Bacon's "methodologies" never gained wide credence or acceptance. William Harvey made sport of them, saying that Bacon wrote of science like a Lord Chancellor. But the logic of the "new life"—that of the dominance of man over all things—was congenial to the mood of the new world and was not challenged until our own times.

The sequence of an improvement in agriculture as a prerequisite to technological progress and the accumulation of capital, so essential to the development of an industrial machine economy, has been clearly expounded by Professor Rostow of the Massachusetts Institute of Technology. It is supported by historic experience. In our own exposition, we sketch a collateral sequence. Man acquired fire, and with it he both increased and improved his foods. More and more of his kind populated the earth. Man learned how to use fire to smelt metals. Out of metals he made superior tools and powerful machines. With machines and fires he harnessed steam. And through them he generated electricity. By means of electricity he loosed the captive energy of the atom.

If we accept Linton's estimate, Man achieved all this in the span of some thirty thousand years (2). But most of the great technological advances were made during the past five to six hundred years.

It was during this latter period that Man seemingly grew utterly insensible to the meaning and interplay of ecology. Man became the wastrel of the earth. Beast, bird, fish, water, air, the woods, soil, and even his own kind became expendable, without account, without remorse, without concern, and all in the pursuit of his mastery over Nature and the earth. True, his was seldom a calculated villainy, or even a deliberate performance. It was a by-product of intentions and purposes that either innately were, or were rationalized as being, good, laudable, and progressive. No one planned and deliberately created those slum areas that were the festering sores of the industrial cities of Europe and America. But they did come into being and some remain to this very day. No one but "conditions" compelled men, women and children to work long hours, under taxing and unhygienic circumstances. But they did, and the effects of these experiences, these ecological disruptions, also remain.

It may seem odd to picture Man as an ecological unit, or the relation of man to man as an ecological dynamic. But that is only because we are accustomed to think of Man as the pinnacle of creation, and all the rest as his *to do with,* a conceit initially propounded in the Book of Genesis (Chap. I, v. 26). But only to himself is Man the pinnacle of creation. Nature knew and seemingly "cared" for other creatures long before Man emerged on earth, and Nature is likely to continue to care for other creatures long after Man has disappeared from the face of the earth—unless, of course, the earth itself, together with Man, has been reduced to primal matter and energy in some atomic holocaust.

Though this is a dismal prospect, it need not, and should not, be taken as earnest prophecy. For in all this exposition, we have been concerned with Western Man, and more particularly with Europe. We have followed *his* history, *his* developments. But there are also vast areas of the East and of Africa, which have not yet been wholly corrupted by Western technological culture. There are still peoples who eschew killing animals, and who, when their plough scores the earth, pray for forgiveness. These people are *not* insensible to the meaning of ecology.

This too is an excursus. Let me return then to the main thread of my theme. Man has wantonly depleted the earth and all that lives on it to serve his purposes and his conceits. He has thereby disturbed the ecology (the better term is the ecosystem) to the detriment of all this system embraces, including Man himself. Man has upset "the accord set up by Zeus" and has, like Prometheus, suffered the wrath of Zeus. Until, like Prometheus of later versions, he is redeemed, Man will continue to suffer, until he too redeems himself. How? Whence may come his redemption? In answer let me quote Paul B. Sears: "Change in the ecosystem of which Man is part is inevitable, since this system is a process, and he is inevitably affected by such changes. On the whole, those changes which are natural (i.e., not due to his interference) take place on a scale and at a rate which is not disastrous to him. While some of his activities may regulate and utilize these changes to his benefit, more of them serve to accelerate the rate and widen the scope of natural changes in ways that lower the potential of the environment to sustain him. For such effects man is responsible, and where responsibility enters so do ethical problems . . .

"Through science, Man now has the means to be aware of change and its effects and the ways in which his cultural values and behavior should be modified to insure their own preservation. Whether we consider ethics to be enlightened self-interest, the greatest good for the greatest number, ultimate good rather than present benefit, or Schweitzer's reverence for life, Man's obligation toward environment is equally clear" (14).

Clear also is this, that we begin with science and end with ethics. Ecology essentially is a discipline in science, but it is, as Sauer affirms, also freighted with moral issues and mortal consequences.

And, need we underscore the timeliness of this consideration? Most probably, yes! For in the ordinary we are too dazzled by the technological achievements in present-day life to see the other elements in the setting—much psychological suffering and illness, increasing technological unemployment, a mounting flood of aging persons doomed to dry rot, a pervasive mood of dependency, a feverish quest for security, the loss of meaning in life, work and possessions, and, above all else, the dread of thermonuclear war. The crowd diseases, those that dominated man's thoughts for long—tuberculosis, typhoid, typhus, cholera, in a word, the infectious diseases—have been mastered. Now we become aware of the emotional, psychological, social, economic and cultural ills affecting our society. These ills are no less to be ascribed to distortion of the ecosystem than are the infectious epidemic diseases and the disorders of mass malnutrition. In all this it is most distressing to perceive that those who *are* concerned, and those who either are charged with the responsibility for seeking remedies, as is government, or voluntarily undertake it, as do the schools and universities, pay little or no attention to ecology and seemingly have no sense of the ecosystem and its interactions.

Most lacking in these respects appear to be certain groups of economists and sociologists intensely animated with a zeal to manipulate the world. The economists are zealous to help history attain its destined ends (a Marxist formualtion); the sociologists to correct the patent evils in contemporary social and economic existence. With the best of intentions, both groups pressure the ecosystem in the direction of their persuasions and quite frequently succeed in changing its contours and dynamics. Yet, insofar as they are, and remain, unmindful of the collateral untoward effects of their manipulations, they practice scientific quackery.

These last observations must not, of course, be construed as a plea for a return to the Good Old Days or as a defense of the status quo. Nor have I meant to denigrate the efforts of economists and sociologists.

If mankind is to survive, and I believe it will, even if its Western segment obliterates itself, it will need to learn in time to understand the initial wrath of Zeus. It will then perceive in the punishment of Prometheus not Olympian retribution, but a warning. It will recall that Pandora's Box, after all its afflictions had escaped, still contained hope. It will grasp that *Homo sapiens* and *Homo faber* are dear to Zeus, if they but function within the accord set up by him. Man will then understand what Anaximander meant in the warning: "Things must pay one another the penalty and compensation for their injustices according to the ordinance of time" (15).

Pandora's Box still harbors hope, and we must hope to share in it. Otherwise there is the spectre of Prometheus' doom, so majestically pictured by Aeschylus:

> "Lo, in grim earnest the world
> Is shaken, the roar of thunders
> Reverberates, gleams the red levin
> And whirlwinds lick up the dust.
> All the blasts of the winds leap out
> And meet in tumultuous conflict,
> Confounding the sea and the heavens" (16).

How very reminiscent are these lines of the mushroom cloud that rose one fateful day to darken the horizons of the morrow.

REFERENCES

1. Stewart, O. C. Fire as the first great force employed by man. In: *Man's Role in Changing the Face of the Earth,* W. L. Thomas, Jr., Ed. Chicago: Chicago University Press, 1956, p. 117.
2. Linton, R. & Linton, A. *Man's Way from Cave to Skyscraper.* New York: Harper, 1947, p. 26.
3. Darby, H. C. The clearing of the woodland in Europe. In: *Man's Role in Changing the Face of the Earth,* W. L. Thomas, Jr., Ed. Chicago: Chicago University Press, 1956, p. 191.
4. Boissonnade, P. *Life and Work in Medieval Europe.* London: Routledge, 1927, pp. 72-73.
5. *Ibid.,* p. 229.
6. *Ibid.,* p. 229.
7. *Ibid.,* p. 230.
8. *Ibid.,* pp. 237-38.
9. Curschman, F. *Hungersnote im Mittelalter.* Leipzig, 1900.
10. Collingwood, R. C. *The Idea of Nature.* Oxford: Clarendon Press, 1945, p. 5.
11. Singer, C. *From Magic to Science.* New York: Boni, 1928, p. 110.
12. Fischer, K. *Francis Bacon of Verulam.* London: Longmans, 1857.
13. *Ibid.,* p. 45.
14. Sears, P. B. The process of environmental change by man. In: *Man's Role in Changing the Face of the Earth,* W. L. Thomas, Jr., Ed. Chicago: Chicago University Press, 1956, p. 481.
15. Jaeger, W. *Paideia: The Ideals of Greek Culture,* Vol. I. New York: Oxford University Press, 1945, p. 159.
16. Aeschylus. *Prometheus Bound.* In: *The Complete Greek Drama,* Vol. I, W. J. Oates & E. O'Neill, Jr., Eds. New York: Random House, 1938.

5

Trade Routes and Medicine

What I say here on trade routes and medical education is intended to be both expository and polemical. It is, in other words, an historical exposition with a purpose. It aims not only to advance certain new ideas, but also to controvert certain old ideas on the development of medical knowledge and its diffusion by education.

The old ideas, those which have been crystallized during the past hundred years, and which are current today, are essentially of an evolutionist character. They incorporate and reflect the persuasions of the 19th century evolutionist philosophers and sociologists, of G. F. Hegel, Herbert Spencer, August Comte, and Karl Marx.

These persuasions embrace two distinctive commitments: the first holds that all experience in time follows a distinctive and discernible pattern of progression. Hegel phrased it as a cyclical advance from thesis to antithesis to synthesis, and Spencer as an unending progression from the simple to the complex, and from the homogeneous to the heterogenous.

The second commitment concerns the dynamics of historical or evolutionary progression. There is, it is postulated, an inherent driving force, and an intuitive directional prescience or discretion, which guides and directs the evolutionary progression. The evolutionary scheme is thus pictured as substantively and dynamically self-contained and presided over by a unique entelechy.

In the light of these persuasions, it is easy to understand why the evolutionist philosophers and sociologists inspired, and were partisans of, the *laissez-faire* school of thought, which, in a succinct sense, can be described as maintaining that "Nature knows best."

In a certain sense this was, and still is, a comforting thought. It relieves the top dog from the need to search his soul, and helps to reconcile the underdog to his lower status. But though comforting, the thought is not competent to answer the gnawing question of the individual's role in the evolutionary scheme of things. Is he, the individual, to be a passive creature, lending himself to the portage of the evolutionary process, or is there some active role which is his to play; if the latter, whence is he to draw the requisite guidance as to *what* he is to do, and *how* to do it?

This problem, incidentally, plagues the Marxist-Communist theoreticians. For they are primarily evolutionists, and firmly believe in the inevitable disintegration of the capitalist system and the triumph of communism. Marx forecast the pattern of this distintegration. The dilemma that confronts the Marxists amounts to this: If inevitable, why not wait for the inevitable to occur in inevitable time? Contrariwise, if the inevitable requires the intervention of man, then is it truly inevitable?

Marxists are expert in dialectic contortions, and they meet this paradox with a neat, though not ultimately definitive "solution," which can be phrased thus: The "inevitable" is inherent in, and derives from, the evolutionary pattern. Man is one of the implementing components of that pattern. It lies within the competence of Man to perceive, in an anticipatory sense, the evolutionary pattern and to align himself with it. He thus helps to create "the wave of progress" on whose crest he will, by reward, ride into the promised future.

Of course there is one catch in this neat solution, and that concerns the authenticity of the evolutionary process and of Man's competence to perceive it in an anticipatory perspective. The catch, defined in epistomological and psychological terms, adds up to this: Is there, in effect, an intrinsic evolutionary pattern to be perceived, or is the entirety of evolutionary schematization an imposition upon experience of Man's propensity to organize perception into distinctive patterns?

The issue is of enormous significance; for if it is true, as the philosophical and sociological evolutionists contend, that historical experience is determined by some inherent, transcending, determinate pattern, then Man must indeed be an impotent creature limited to the choice of either conforming to the scheme of things innate and thus surviving for a time, or failing to do so, and suffering in dire consequence what our communist friends so euphemistically term "liquidation." On the other hand, if the evolutionary pattern is taken to be no more than a convenient scheme for organizing data, like the decimal system in arithmetic; if there is nothing inevitable and compelling in the pattern; and if the data of experience could be schematized otherwise, then Man is emancipated to seek his human ends in human terms, and in human ways. He is freed from bondage to the mythical scheme of Nature and its intentions, and at the same time is saddled with responsibilities for the discrete, intelligent management of his human intentions within the realities of Nature.

The pertinence of the aforegoing lies in the fact that during the past hundred years the history of medicine has been schematized on an evolutionary pattern. Medical-historical thinking has been based on a commitment to evolutionary predeterminism.

Fielding H. Garrison, in his preface to Osler's *The Evolution of Modern Medicine,* wrote: "The slow, painful character of the evolution of medicine from the fearsome, superstitious mental complex of primitive man, with his amulets, healing gods, and disease demons, to the ideal of a clear-eyed rationalism, is traced with faith and a serene sense of continuity" (1). Osler, in turn, quoted as a motto to his book a passage from the writings of Walter Moxon. "A golden thread," wrote Moxon, "has run throughout the history of the world, consecutive and continuous, the work of the best men in successive ages. From point to point it still runs, and when near, you feel it as the clear and bright and searchingly irresistible light which Truth throws forth when great minds conceive it" (2). In these two quotations we witness the profession of faith and a serene sense of continuity in that golden thread of Truth that presumptively has run throughout history—still runs from point to point, and bids fair to continue running till time's end.

There is something charming and seductive in these passages, treating as they do of faith, serenity, and effulgent Truth, made manifest in successive instalments. They are reminiscent of the sweet and gullible mood that prevailed in the late years of the 19th Century, and in our own until the rude awakening of 1914. But it is precisely because of that rude awakening and of the even more disruptive and distressing sociocultural experiences that followed in its wake that we are *not* charmed for long, nor effectively seduced. We recognize the naiveté of the faith, the fragility of the serenity, and the tarnish on that golden thread of Truth.

We are likely to be more responsive to the sober affirmation of the wise and learned Castiglioni, who wrote, "He who follows the history of medical thought in its various branches will not find, as has been often and inaccurately stated, the continuous progress of a constantly ascending line. It is with strange interferences and marvelous spirals that this thought progresses from the demonism of the ancients to the suggestive healing of our times, from Biblical organ therapy to recent glandular doctrines, from the humoral pathology of Hippocrates to modern immunology" (3). "The changing succession of errors and victories," Castiglioni affirms, "constitute the very essence of our history, which leads us, by paths that are sometimes luminous and at other times barely discernible, to laws that today seem impregnable and yesterday were dogmas, to hypotheses that perhaps tomorrow will be truths" (4).

In this pungent passage Castiglioni juxtaposes not errors with truths, but errors and victories. He clearly shies away from identifying effectiveness with truth. He is content to equate effectiveness with victory. The history of medicine thus mirrors neither a mystical revelation of absolute Truth nor the evolutionary emergence of an indwelling potential of perfectibility.

Medical history lends itself to being chronicled, but not in such wise as to suggest that it is the log of an autonomy in momentum and direction. The authentic history of medicine is effectively an abstraction and refinement of given segments of experience drawn from the larger history of different peoples in different times and places. These segments relate in especial ways to the health of people, to the selection, training, and practices of their healers, to the beliefs and rationalizations concerning health and sickness shared in given times and places by the peoples and their healers.

Medical history thus understood has no primary existence of its own. It is derivative, like the history of Architecture or of Military Science, from the larger embracive history of Man. It carries within its own chronicles the witness of the determinants which shaped the larger destinies of mankind.

I will illustrate and support this contention with an "exposition" on the relation of trade routes to medicine and to medical education. The term "exposition" is perhaps somewhat pretentious—"excursus" would be more appropriate, for I shall offer no more than a general statement, and some specific instances by way of illustration.

It can be validly affirmed that medicine as a profession, the pursuit of the science of medicine, and medical education are prone to prosper, as the people prosper, and most notably where they prosper most. Conversely, as a people or a locus declines in prosperity, so does the medicine of that place and that people.

Historically, human prosperity is related to trade and commerce. Both, trade and commerce, attest to the emergence of human existence above the subsistence level and are in themselves an indication of a higher cultural development. It is not by happenstance then that, as one scans the trade routes of times past, that is, of antiquity and down the ages, one perceives that on land at given points, and by sea at given ports, trade routes stretch between the loci of great cities in many of which important medical centers developed. In Greek antiquity it was Cnossos, Mycenae, Corinth, Megara, Athens, Samos, Cos, and Rhodes. Later it was Rome, with farflung outposts spreading to all points of the compass. The lanes of commerce crisscrossed the Mediterranean and reached even the farthermost points of the ancient world—Kitai (China) and the fabulous Indies.

Fascinating is the historic play of fortune that made some coastal cities preeminent for a time and thereafter reduced them to nothingness, favoring others in their stead. This seeming pattern of Fortune's fickleness is, in effect, a tracery of the lines of conflict among the early historic peoples for the possession of land, colonies, and trade.

The rise of the *polis,* the city, favored the development of the crafts, and their produce was, in time, exchanged for that of other regions and cities. Thus it was that trade developed, mediated by seafarers, merchants, and markets. Thus, too, was the ground laid for wars in endless succession, even unto our own times. As trade prospered, market cities grew in population and wealth, and formed the nodal points of cultural development. When the fortunes of war shifted, the fortunes of cities were also likely to change, so that what was for a time a prosperous center of commerce and culture, could in a short time become a wasteland. And some among the cities that once prospered and then declined were, in their heyday, significant and even preeminent medical centers.

The destinies of individual market cities must not, however, divert us from the larger view of the shifting itineraries of trade routes, and the consequent emergence of new city centers that prospered in trade and grew in cultural dimensions.

There is some convenience in speaking of the city center that stood forth, historically, in commerce or culture. The identification of, say, Epidaurus, Cos, Athens, or Alexandria, is easy. But in each instance the city refers to a people, and to that people's distinctive cultural orientation. Hence, it is to be appreciated that the rise and fall of city centers, and the coincident shift in trade routes, favored the emergence of new cultural components; these, in turn, affected and altered both commerce and culture.

These changes were primarily geographical, but they were also cultural. The new city centers, quite like the preceding ones, fostered cultural developments, but somewhat discontinuously, that is, in the bias and with the imprint of their own cultural orientations.

Since medicine is a component of culture, it was perforce affected by the shifting accents of the different cultural orientations of the different city centers in which it was cultivated. The history of medicine thus reflects the discontinuity that characterizes the embracive history of human experience and of human culture.

In the argument propounded, trade and commerce have been conjoined with culture in general and medicine in particular, in a manner so intimate as to suggest Siamese twins. It would be easy, though entirely erroneous, to draw from this conclusion that what is here propounded is a theory of the economic determinism of medicine. The relation between trade, commerce, and culture (medicine included) is relational but not causative. It is Man who develops production, commerce, and trade. It is Man's manipulation of these processes that reflexly affects culture. The processes do not of themselves have any autonomous and overriding influence.

But history does attest that the decline of production, trade and commerce causes a lag, and at times a regression in cultural development. Such was the effect upon the Roman realm of the Arabian conquests in the 7th century. "From the 7th to the 11th century Islam was incontestably the master of the Mediterranean," wrote Henry Pirenne. "Three fourths of the littoral of this sea, hitherto the common center of European Civilization, now belonged to Islam" (5). "In the second half of the 7th Century all trade ceased on the shores of the Western Mediterranean" (6).

"The most important fact, from the social point of view, of the period extending from the Muslim invasions of the Carolingian epoch was the rapid reduction, and in the end, the all but complete disappearance, of the urban population" (7).

From the 8th century onwards, Europe existed for three hundred years without any intercourse with the countries overseas. The inevitable consequence was an almost complete cessation of trade, and, apart from a few local industries, such as weaving of cloth, which still survived in Flanders, there was an almost total failure of industrial activity, and money no longer circulated.

The decline of the West had, in effect, commenced some centuries before the time of Mohammed, but his followers hastened its culmination. "The fall of the Roman Empire of the West," wrote Castiglioni, "marks a period of arrest in the history of (Western) civilization. Rigidified in a system of formulas and dominated by mysticism, medicine was forced to exist in a state of scholastic dogmatism, in which it is difficult to find any animating ideas" (8).

From this time until the time of the Renaissance, not Europe but the lands of the Caliphates sustained and furthered the cultures of antiquity.

They advanced the art, the science, and the teaching of medicine. The trade routes that once led Westward now were *Eastward* bent. The Arabs were master merchants. "From India they imported sugar cane into Sicily and Africa, rice into Sicily and Spain . . ., and cotton into Sicily and Africa; they acclimatized in Asia the manufacture of silk, which they learned from the Chinese; and from the Chinese also they learned the use and manufacture of paper . . .; and from China they imported the magnetic compass" (9).

During this period, the non-Islamic remnants of Europe, in contrast, suffered impoverishment and deprivation. Papyrus, so vital to commerce, communication, and culture, disappeared, and spices, too, for they came in the same vessels. The wine of Gaza could not be had, and oil was no longer imported from Africa. Parchment replaced papyrus, and wax candle, the oil lamp. The use of silk became almost unknown, and gold became a rarity.

The Arabs were also good sailors. They constructed the ports of Cairo, Tunis, and Kairouan, and these served as "the *ètapes* of a commerce which circulated from the Straits of Gibraltar to the Indian Ocean, through the Egyptian ports, which were in communication with the Red Sea, and the Syrian ports, which gave access to the Caravan route to Baghdad and the Persian Gulf" (10).

In Christian Europe, as Castiglioni observed, medicine existed in a state of scholastic dogmatism, devoid of any animating ideas.

The great schools were now not in Athens, or Rome, but in Baghdad, Samarkand, Ispahan, and Damascus. In these academies, pupils from all parts received their instruction, a little in all sciences, but especially in theology, philosophy, and medicine. In Spain, too, the Islamic influence was witnessed in the rise of splendid and flourishing schools in Cordova, Seville, Toledo, and Murcia.

"The Arabs," Castiglioni affirms, "inherited all the medical partrimony of the past and became the faithful guardians of ancient medicine. When they and their relations disappeared from the theatre of their great exploits, and the fall of the Arabian domination of Spain marked the end of this historic period, the traces that they left were so remarkable that they remain highly significant of the role that the Arabs played in the history of civilization and of medicine" (11).

The Arabs were for long the teachers of the European medical novitiates. The works of Avicenna were read, together with those of Galen, far into the 16th Century, and as Puschmann affirms, Rhazes, Ali-Abbas,

Abulkasem, and Averroes. In addition, Maimonides, Ibn El-Beithar, Oseibia, deserve to be counted among the great men in medicine (12).

The Arabs, who overwhelmed the Christian West in the 7th century, sought in the 10th Century to live beside it in peace. The capture of Taormina in 902 marked the last advance of Islam in the West. Islam was now willing to enjoy, rather than eager to extend, its domain. But the Christian West was not of like mind. At first, sporaidcally in Spain, and later in larger, more aggressive and better organized offensives, the Mussulman was pushed back and ultimately expelled from Europe. Granada was Islam's last stronghold, and it was reconquered by the Catholic Princes in 1492.

The Christian West that was dismally overwhelmed in the 8th century, and remained disorganized for close to three hundred years thereafter, did in the meantime recover a measure of its organic unity. By the end of the 12th century, Europe had not only recovered from the social and economic disorganization which had made it an easy prey to Islamic aggression, but, in fact, fashioned a new and superior socioeconomic order—that of the merchant-adventurer.

Industry came into being, fostered by and fostering commerce. Beginning with the 11th century there developed a new type of merchant city, extending beyond and about the older cities. These were enlarged communities, fortified by moats, thick walls, and ramparts. They were "the nouveau-bourg," or "faubourg," and those who dwelt in them came to be known as the *"bourgeois."*

Driven off the Mediterranean by the Mussulman, and isolated from the East in the 7th century, Europe turned to the lands beyond the Rhine and the shores of the North Sea. Then, when commerce was revived in the 11th century, it was, perforce, carried on, not as formerly by sea, but almost entirely over land routes. In the past the great merchant cities were almost all seaports. Now many of them were literally landlocked.

Now the highways and caravan routes were traveled by merchant adventurers, banded together into trade groups, known as Hanses. Initially, these groups of merchant adventurers were loosely organized for mutual protection against highwaymen and robbers, and at times, too, for joint commercial enterprises, pooling their individual moneys for some common deal of large magnitude. Later, the Hanses became stable and powerful trade organizations, centered in given cities, and federated in leagues that embraced the greater part of Europe.

Commerce encouraged trade and productivity, and also—learning. Commerce makes literacy one of its basic requisites. It fosters the keeping of books, of records, and accounts. It entails correspondence, contracts, and, be it noted also, litigation; hence, it is a "patron" of the law. As for medicine, its effects are multiplex.

Scanning the trade routes, both maritime and overland, that developed in Europe following the revival of trade and commerce, we can perceive that they are dotted with what, in time, came to be major university cities. In a number of these universities the study of medicine was cultivated preeminently.

The Italian cities, Bologna, Padua, Florence, Perugia, to name but a few, were among the earliest to establish universities. France and Spain were not tardy. Indeed, in terms of simple chronology, Paris predates Bologna, and Montpellier, Padua. Northern Italy, however, was the more advanced industrially and commercially. In the 13th century, Siena and Florence were the banking centers of Europe, and remained such until the 15th century. The Florentine weavers were world famous as artists and craftsmen even in the 13th century.

Commercial activity was initially—that is, in the 13th and 14th centuries—most intense in Northern Italy and Southern Europe, and then extended to the more distant regions, North, West and East, and one can perceive a corresponding "transmigration" of academic intensity. The 14th century witnessed the foundation of universities in Prague, Cracow, Vienna, and Cologne. The universities of Ingolstadt, Basel, and Budapest were founded in the 15th century; Leyden, Edinburgh, Strasbourg, Gottingen follow in sequence.

Neither the extension of commerce nor the foundation of universities follows a neat pattern, and they are not *pari passu.* Such a premise is no part of my argument. What is relevant to my exposition is the evident and vital relationship of commercial vitality to academic pursuits in general, and to the development of medical centers for service and education at nodal points in the prospering regions. This is patent, historically, in that those regions which once prospered economically and then regressed do not retain the academic preeminence they may have attained in the times of their prosperity. Again, regions that once were backward, on attaining prosperity are also likely to acquire competences in the realm of learning and science.

The histories of Egypt and Greece, of Byzantium, and of the Islamic lands attest to the first, and those of Germany, France, and Russia to the second instance of the given historical generalization.

I have referred to this historical generalization as "patent." And so it appears. But it also embraces a recondite factor, one that is not patent, and one that is at the very vital core of my argument. In a sense this recondite factor is contrapuntal to my generalization, for it postulates that not all trade routes are "equal"—that it is not of *little* consequence *what* seas or lands the routes traverse, nor *which* peoples ply the routes and pursue the trades. Furthermore, if these be matters of consequence, as I am sure they are, then what derives from them must likewise be different. Neither commerce nor trade is taken over in pristine form, nor with them their associated cultures. Each people in each geographic locus imprints its distinctive features upon whatever it takes over or develops.

Latin is the matrix of French, Italian, Spanish, and Portuguese, and yet how much they do differ, one language from the others. The medicine the Arabs learned from their Nestorian teachers they transmuted, and when they brought it back to the West by way of the Sicilian Isle and Salerno, it was both less and more than they had learned. It was different!

I am sure that it must sound heretical, yet I would affirm that different also is the medicine of the Germanic peoples, the Gauls, the Franks, the Norsemen, the Slavs, the Iberians, not in primitive or even prehistoric times, but rather in recent times, as these peoples have had the opportunity to cultivate medicine in their respective spheres of economic and cultural influence.

Thus, medicine which seemingly has an historic continuity, is experientially discontinuous. The unity, consistency, or congruity that we may perceive in its past, by viewing its emergence, is of our own projection. The data of experience can be added in different ways to yield different summations.

But here it may be asked, granted that it be so, what profit is there in adding the data of historic experience in different ways to yield different summations? It must, however, be clear that the granting of this possibility is itself significant. It renders historical study mobile and plastic rather than rigid and determinate. History is thus conceivable as the unrolling of adventure, rather than as the fulfillment of predetermined ends. Furthermore, it emancipates and enfranchises the individual. Now he has an historic role to play, that is, he can influence rather than merely fulfill history.

All of this has an intimate bearing on medicine and medical education. As we have observed, the common belief is that medicine has "emerged" in an evolutionary and consistently progressive manner from the days of Hippocrates, the Father of Medicine. Time and experience have sharpened the physician's perceptions and have extended and deepened his knowledge of the human organism, and of its operations in health and disease. Medical education has perforce experienced an equivalent development and has been similarly broadened, deepened, and refined. The history of medicine, and of medical education, thus reviewed, cannot but be viewed enthusiastically as a triumphant march. And in this perspective, it cannot but be anticipated that the "triumphant march" will continue—being carried forward by its own momentum and directed by its own insights which have grown ever brighter with the passing of the centuries. There is, accordingly, prevalent a sense of security and contentment, an optimistic expectation of future good, inspired by this perception of the history of medicine.

But, as I have attempted to show, this historic perception is fictional. Neither medicine nor medical education has emerged in any consistently evolutionary or progressive manner. Medicine and medical education are tied in with the changing destinies of peoples and places, so neatly mirrored in their trades, commerce, and trade routes. The destinies of peoples have been checkered, and so, too, has been the history of medicine and of medical education. But checkered history is history, nonetheless, and even if lacking in consistency, it can bear witness to some orders of change that enhance those qualities of being which render human existence civilized and cultured. To insist that history is not consistent is not to totally deny the possibilities of change toward the humanly preferable.

But to deny that history is consistent and evolutionary in a deterministic pattern is also to regain some prerogatives of initiative for the individual. If the history of medicine and of medical education reflect not a consistent progression but the vicarious play of blind fortune, then Man, too, can enter the play of forces, and deliberately, that is thoughtfully, seek to mold the patterns of medicine and medical education of his own perceptions of what they can and need be.

It may, however, be asked, is not this precisely what is now being done in scores of institutions by numerous study and curriculum committees and commissions?

In a given sense, in terms of effort, yes! But the framework of these deliberations, their intellectual and historical orientation, is usually not of the order I intend. They are, perhaps, without even being aware of it, committed to the thesis of the evolutionary, consistently progressive development of medicine. In such a commitment, the prerogatives of initiative are much constrained. Initiative and originality too easily become—deviation!

This is too large a subject to argue in detail here. But I would submit that the current medical curriculum to a very large extent, and step by step, recapitulates in four years the past four hundred years in the development of medical knowledge.

Perhaps if we undertook to add the data of historic experience in a different way, we might gain a different summation, one more pertinent to our current problems and needs.*

But that is not the note on which I want to end. I want rather to offer an "apologia" for my presentation and for this intention I shall borrow the words of Diez del Corral, who in his superb work *The Rape of Europe* affirms: "The depth of the future is proportionatte to the depth of the awareness of the past" (13). And he quotes Sartre, who wrote "History is not characterized by change, nor by the pure and simple action of the past: it is defined by the intentional resumption of the past by the present."

The history of Europe, in which we share, is divided into three Ages: the Ancient, the Medieval, and that Age, now terminal, which was born with the Renaissance. We are on the brink of a fourth Age! Our accustomed orientations do not and will not do; they suited the past—not the future. It is high time that we intentionally "resume" the past in the present—review the data of the past in the perspectives of the present. This is what I have endeavored to do.

REFERENCES

1. Osler, W. *The Evolution of Modern Medicine.* New Haven: Yale University Press, 1921, p. xiv.
2. Moxon, W. *Philocereus Sevrilis and Other Papers.* London: Low, 1887, p. 4.
3. Castiglioni, A. *A History of Medicine.* New York: Knopf, 1947, p. 3.
4. *Ibid.*, p. 5.
5. Pirenne, H. *A History of Europe.* New York: University Book Pub., 1955, p. 48.
6. *Ibid.*, p. 72.
7. *Ibid.*, p. 94.
8. Castiglioni, A. *Op. cit.*, p. 258.
9. Pirenne, H. *Op. cit.*, p. 49.
10. *Ibid.*, pp. 49, 50.
11. Castiglioni, A. *Op. cit.*, p. 261.
12. Puschmann, T. *Geschichte des Medizinischen Unterrichts.* Leipzig: Veit & Comp., 1889, pp. 138, 201-279.
13. Diez del Corral, L. *The Rape of Europe.* New York: Macmillan, 1959.

---

* Lest I be suspected of indulging in the fatuous satisfaction of "urging the other mouse to bell the cat," let me refer to my own efforts to reassess the data of experience and gain a different summation, published as *The Meaning of Social Medicine,* Harvard University Press, Cambridge, Mass., 1954.

6

Diagnosis in Historical Perspective

In 1836, the Boylston Medical Committee of Harvard University advanced as a prize thesis the question, "How far are the external means of exploring the condition of the internal organs to be considered useful and important in medical practice?"

Of the dissertations submitted, the best was adjudged to be one bearing the motto *Inter labores et taedia.* When the sealed envelope accompanying this dissertation was opened, the name found therein was that of Oliver Wendell Holmes. He was then 27 years of age.

Holmes was, therefore, awarded first prize. But two other essays were also considered highly meritorious, and two added awards were made, to Dr. Robert W. Haxall (1802-72) of Richmond, Virginia, and to Dr. Luther Vose Bell (1806-62) of Derry, New Hampshire.

These essays were thought so valuable that the Massachusetts Medical Society authorized their publication in book form (1) and their gratuitous distribution to "each fellow of the Society and to every other respectable physician in Massachusetts." In these three essays we find a clear representation of *diagnosis* as it was understood and practiced nearly a century and a half ago.

Of the three, the ablest essay appears to be that of Bell, while Haxall's contribution is hardly noteworthy. Holmes' dissertation, as is to be expected, has a superior literary quality, but it lacks the scholarly foundation and the breadth of vision that distinguishes Dr. Bell's contribution.

There is a refreshing and entirely modern spirit in Bell's words. "Symptoms," he wrote, ". . . are not disease; they are merely the language, the signs; the appreciable evidence of some internal change which is invisible to our senses in a great degree during life, and the presumed effects of which are in part manifested after death."

Symptoms are divided by Bell into two groups, one vital or physiological, the second, physical. Among the vital symptoms, he lists the pulse, the seat of suffering, the bodily expression, and the patient's recitation of the history of his disorder.

"The symptoms of disease," Bell wrote, "are addressed to various, indeed, it may now be said, to the entire circle of our external senses." He lists then the eye, the ear, the sense of smell, and the sense of taste, citing as an instance of how taste may be employed in the diagnosis of "the one fatal and highly interesting disease . . . diabetes mellitus."

Bell then singles out the sense of hearing "once scarcely available to any extent in the healing art" and devotes the remaining portion of his dissertation to the inventions which had produced "results most extraordinary, unequivocal, and useful." The inventions he refers to are thoracic percussion, and auscultation.

Holmes' essay begins with a bold attack on the question set. Inspection, mensuration, palpation, auscultation, percussion and succussion are listed as the external means by which the condition of the internal organs may be determined.

As to auscultation, it is gratifying to find the author of the Satirical Stethoscope Song writing in a vein faintly suggestive of surprise and indignation at the indifference shown to Laennec and his invention. "The new methods of direct exploration," Holmes wrote, "can only be said to have been before the English and American public for the space of fifteen years. It is to be remembered that in the very city where they originated, the discoveries of Laennec were not at once received without opposition. Thus, in the first edition of the *Dictionary of Medicine,* in twenty-one volumes, the author of the article Auscultation estimated so very moderately the importance of the new method of exploration that after reading it one might have been tempted to throw the stethoscope in the receptacle which holds the scala of Hippocrates and the balance of Sanctorius."

The warrant for dwelling at such length on the Boylston Committee prize thesis of 1836 appears to me to be the intrinsic interest of the question proposed and of the prize essays submitted. Here we find authentication for the words of the well known French clinician, Charles Achard, who wrote:

> At the beginning of the nineteenth century, the clinician observed studiously the "facies," the general aspect, and the constitutional

> habitus (of the patient); he examined the tongue, the mirror of the stomach; he palpated the pulse (*tâtait le pouls*), gaged the temperature of the skin with his hand, and observed the gross characteristics of the urine, of the excreta (*des Selles*) and of the expectorants. He practiced palpation—"*et le toucher*" (3).*

These representations afford us a base from which to set out in our review of the development of diagnosis. They afford us a norm by which we can gauge the progress made during the past century. Cleaving to the core of our matter, let us set in apposition to the foregoing the description of the diagnostic instruments and procedures available to the medical man at the beginning of the 20th century. I quote from an address delivered in 1916 by Lewellys F. Barker, entitled "The Development of the Science of Diagnosis" (4). The fourth year medical student or the young intern, Dr. Barker said, is able to "inspect, to percuss, to auscultate, to make a bacterial culture or a Wasserman test, to measure systolic and diastolic blood pressure, to pass a stomach tube, to do a phenolphthalein test, to make a differential count of the white blood corpuscles, to study roentgenograms, to examine eyegrounds, to test reflexes, to do lumbar punctures, to titrate glucose—and the like."

That was spoken in 1916, and the list is already impressive. To catalogue the instrumentalities and diagnostic procedures added to it since that date would prove a trying task and unprofitable here. For even my cursory review indicates that the science of diagnosis, as we know it and practice it today, is of very recent origin. It is little more than a century old. It is still a young science, experiencing the growth spurts of juvenility.

Instead of describing the diagnostic armamentarium, I want to discuss the non-instrumental aspects of diagnosis. For to diagnose is to perform a function and that function cannot be defined in terms of the instruments employed or of the techniques pursued.

Oddly, very few, even among those who have written text books on diagnosis, have attempted to define its nature, its quality, and its ultimate objectives. In a search of the literature (not too exhaustive, I must confess), I found but one author who boldly faces the question. Ludolph

---

* The essays of Holmes and Bell also echo the words of S. Weir Mitchell (1830-1914), whom Garrison titles the historian of instrumental precision in medicine. Mitchell wrote, "When I was a lad, there were then alive men who could recall when what a patient said, and the physician saw and felt, were all that a case of disease had to tell him."

Krehl (5) both sets and answers the question, "Was sollen und wollen wir diagnostizieren? Was gehort zu Diagnose?" In answer, he wrote:

> It (i.e. diagnosis) is the summation of all that deviates from the normal in a sickly body. This involves much more than is commonly thought. We need to know both the kind and degree of functional disturbance affecting an organ-system. We must clearly determine the underlying histopathological and chemical changes. Finally, we must seek to establish the cause of illness, and also the collateral effects of the disorder upon the organs not immediately involved. In other words, everything that is abnormal must be summed up in the diagnosis in such wise that all the signs and symptoms are accounted for and integrated. All of this must be established relative to a given person with definite psychological and physical endowments who lives under particular circumstances and in a given milieu. *Das endziel der diagnose*—the ultimate objective of diagnosis—is to recognize and to determine *welchen einfluss die krankheit auf diesen einen Menschen hat.* Precisely what effect the illness has on this singular person."

Contrast with this rather involved, but in many respects competent, definition of diagnosis that, or rather those, given by the dictionary. The dictionary gives the philology of the term as being, *dia* = apart + *gnosis* = knowledge. It proceeds to define diagnosis as: 1) the art of distinguishing one disease from another; 2) the determination of the nature of a case of disease. Then we come upon the variety of terms prefixed to diagnosis to form compounds—such as biological, clinical, differential and direct diagnosis; diagnosis by exclusion, group diagnosis, and laboratory diagnosis; pathological, physical, regional roentgen, and serum diagnosis; and last, but not least, tentative diagnosis.

In this contrast we see the fundamental problem of diagnosis. This problem troubled Hippocrates, and stirred his passions. It continues to agitate the best of our medical contemporaries, for it lies at the very core of our professional competence. We must resolve whether diagnosis is, as the dictionary maintains, "the art of distinguishing one disease from another," or as Krehl (quoted only as prototype) contends, the summation of all that deviates from the normal in a sick individual of definite psychological and physical endowments living under particular circumstances in a given milieu.

I believe it will be granted that diagnosis as it is practiced today more often conforms to its dictionary definition than to the other. Medical history, on the other hand, reveals that the best clinicians have understood and practiced diagnosis in its broadest encompassments.

This matter is of no small moment. Nosology, the classification of disease, is today a highly developed science. Only a little less well developed is the science of specific and near specific therapy. Between the two, it would seem, all medical knowledge is confined. On the other hand, time and time again we hear some strident, some commanding, some pleading voice raised in protest, contending that our crystallized nosology hampers no less than it aids the understanding of morbid processes, that our specific and near specific therapies, useful as they are in dealing with the emergency episodes in disease, distract us from the more fundamental and effective treatment and correction of disease. This is an old complaint. We find it in Hippocrates. In *Ancient Medicine* it is written:

> All who, on attempting to speak or to write on medicine, have assumed for themselves a postulate as a basis for their discussion—heat, cold, moisture, dryness, or anything else that they may fancy—who narrow down the causal principles of diseases and of death among men, and make it the same in all cases, postulating one thing or two, all these obviously blunder in many points even of their statements, but they are most open to censure because they blunder in what is an art, and one which all men use on the most important occasions, and give the greatest honors to the good craftsmen and practitioners in it (6).

If we substitute for the terms "heat, cold, moisture, dryness" their present-day equivalents which "narrow down the causal principle of diseases and death among men, and make it the same in all cases, postulating one thing or two," we find Hippocrates' arguments and censures as valid today as when first expounded, twenty-four hundred years ago.

At the time of Hippocrates, there existed two dominant schools of medical thought and practice, that of Cos, to which Hippocrates belonged, and that of Cnidus, of which (Galen tells us) the chief physician, was Euryphon.

Between the schools of Cos and Cnidus there were wide divergences in thought and practice. The Cnidians were "long on diagnosis and short on therapy." They classified diseases according to numerous divisions and subdivisions, taking as their basis minute variations and symptoms. Hippocrates and the Coan physicians were little preoccupied with the minutia of diagnosis. In the words of W. H. S. Jones—the English translator of Hippocrates—the Coan physician "held that it was impossible to decide with certainty when a variation in the symptoms constituted a different disease, and he blamed the Cnidian physicians for multiplying types by assigning essential importance to accidental details. He attached far less value to diagnosis than he did to what may perhaps be called general pathology of morbid conditions, in particular of acute diseases. In all these diseases, according to Hippocrates, there are symptoms, or combinations of symptoms, which point to certain consequences in either the near or the remote future. In other words there is a common element, of which can be written a common medical history" (7).

Jones is partial to the Cnidian school. He somewhat excuses what he considers to be the Hippocratic limitations, in explaining that "it must be remembered that the means of treatment available to Hippocrates were few in number. The most he could do was to hinder Nature as little as possible in her efforts to expel a disease, and to assuage pain as far as the limited knowledge of the time permitted."

"To a certain extent," Jones writes, "this view is correct; in the Hippocratic age little could be done for patients suffering from acute diseases except to keep them warm and comfortable and to restrict their diet. Yet we must always remember that 'general' pathology really does not exist, and that any prognosis based upon it must be very uncertain indeed."

Littré, the illustrious French translator of Hippocrates, is also much intrigued by this divergence between the schools of Cos and Cnidus. He does not, however, share the opinions of Jones. In vigorous language, he expounds the differences between Cos and Cnidus and emphatically registers his sympathy with the school of Hippocrates.

> The basic principle of the method of Cos is prognosis. That is to say, a prepondering study of the different aspects of the general condition.
>
> The basic principle of the method of Cnidian physicians is their failure to be concerned with the issue and the development of the malady and in their being content most of the time with the description of symptoms and of incidentals. It is for Hippocrates, an accepted and specifically expressed injunction that one should learn from the regimen of men while they are as yet in health. Hippocrates attacks the Cnidian physicians and reproaches them for being too much concerned with the details of the maladies, for failing to apply even that concern in their therapy, and for prescribing too few remedies. That which Hippocrates desires above all is a substitution for the *hypothesis,* the study of the living being (*tou anthropon*) of the reality (*tou eontos*), and the study of the manner which the body reacts (*se comporte*) in regard to everything (8).

I must draw attention to a sentence quoted from Jones, for it touches the heart of the matter. Jones wrote: "Yet we must always remember that 'general' pathology really does not exist and that any prognosis based upon it must be very uncertain indeed" (9).

In these words, Jones echoes the high hopes and the pretensions of the histopathologists, first promulgated by Virchow and supported since his time by many pathologists. Experience and increasing knowledge have invalidated these pretensions and dissipated these hopes. We have come to recognize that pathological reactions are, to use scholastic terms, more universal than particular. The reverse conviction has given rise to numerous blunders and mountainous but sterile labors.*

This matter of "general" pathology was concisely summed up by Lorenz S. Michaëlis. "What we can see on a slide," wrote Michaëlis, "are the responses of cells and tissues to aetiological factors. The number of these (aetiological) factors is almost unlimited, but the variety of responses is not. The number of different changes a cell or a tissue can undergo is very small indeed. And furthermore, each kind of cell or tissue has to rely on its own specific and limited choice of responses to the great variety of factors able to provoke a response" (10).

What has been said of pathology holds equally true of symptomatology. Since Johannes Müller formulated the law of specific physiological response, we have known that it is impossible to infer from the physiological response the nature of the stimulus provoking it. There is then, as Hippocrates maintained, a general pathology and a general symptomatology, both of which serve best as the foundation of diagnosis.

Actually, Hippocrates did not disparage the worth and usefulness of the particular. His *Aphorisms* are in themselves but a precious collection of particulars. What he contended, and I echo his words, was that the particular becomes animate only in the general; that without the matrix of the larger concept, without the regard to the living being and to the reality the particular is likely to be sterile, delusive, and fallacious.

---

* We need only recall the fate of Villemin's brilliant demonstration of the communicability of tuberculosis, which was discredited by Clark, Sanderson, Cohnheimer, B. Frankel, Talma, and M. Wolff. Because these men were able to produce tubercles in animals by inoculating them with a variety of innocuous and miscellaneous substances, they argued against the communicability of tuberculosis. Tubercle formation, as a non-specific tissue response to foreign body invasion, was recognized only after much controversy and many labors. The tuberculosis tubercle was then understood to be a complex of tissue reactions, each non-specific in itself but forming in combination a unique pattern. Thus the tubercle itself is a foreign body reaction; the central necrosis or causation is the effect of the noxious toxins of the tubercle bacillus upon the proximal cells.

This deep conviction has been shared by the best of clinicians in all the ages. It was stoutly defended by Galen and by Sydenham. We find it elaborated with fine scholarship and deep sincerity by William A. White, whose excellent book, *The Meaning of Disease,* is regrettably none too well known to the medical profession (11).

We observe, then, that since the days of Hippocrates "to diagnose" has meant to perform one or the other of two distinctly different functions. To one group it has meant the definition of a disease as a definite and distinct entity. Such was the meaning of diagnosis to the Cnidian school. Such is the more common understanding and practice of diagnosis today. To the other group, the school of Cos, the Hippocratic group, "to diagnose" meant to define a clinical problem in terms of the individual affected, to be solved therapeutically.

This interpretation of diagnosis is enlisting the interest and support of a mounting number of clinicians. In Europe, previous to the outbreak of World War II, there was an organized movement in this direction that went by the name of Neo-Hippocratism.

To those not steeped in these matters, it may seem that the distinctions drawn between diagnosis as the definition of a disease entity and diagnosis as the definition of a clinical problem affecting a given individual to be solved therapeutically is either much ado about little or merely an exercise in dialectics. Such an impression, however, can be promptly dissipated by considering what is implied in the two distinctly different conceptions of the function of diagnosis.

To diagnose a disease as a distinct entity is a more primitive function. It requires but a moderate mental discipline. It can frequently be accomplished by using inanimate instruments. It offers only a narrow and none too stable foundation for effective therapy.

Diagnosis as definition of disease entities predominates when and where physiological knowledge and physiological thinking are lowest.

Diagnosis practiced as the definition of a clinical problem affecting a given individual, to be solved therapeutically, is by far the superior and more difficult function. It is rooted in physiology. It flourishes when and where physiological knowledge and physiological thinking are in the ascendant.

In the emphasis on physiology, we have a clue to the intriguing problem as to why Hippocratic diagnosis differs so radically from diagnosis as we know it today and why there is current among us a revival of the Hippocratic practice. Hippocratic medicine was essentially physiological medicine, and today physiology dominates medical science once again.

Hippocratic physiology was empirical; present day physiology is biochemical. But mark this, both Hippocratic and present day physiology are biological—that is, essentially concerned with the body as a living organism. This type of physiology is distinct from the physiology of the test tube and dissection table, which was cultivated from the 17th to the beginning of the 20th century.* The Hippocratic physician studied man in his environment during health and illness. He noted the factors in diet and environment (airs, waters, and places), rest and exercise which in essence is physiological medicine. It permeates the Hippocratic Corpus and, be it noted, had a long-lasting effect on medicine, even down to the time of the Salernian School, as may be seen in the Regimen of Salerno.

The empirical physiology of Hippocrates was in the 17th century challenged by Sanctorius and by William Harvey. The works of neither Sanctorius nor Harvey had any effect upon the thinking or activities of their medical contemporaries. But with them there was initiated the new science of physiology, one that discredited the old—but one that was of itself unable to give to medicine a supportive framework of theory and fact. We must bear in mind the great confusion, the babble of tongues that filled the medical world from the time of Sydenham until the middle of the 19th century. Garrison labels the 17th century the Age of Individual Scientific Medicine, and the 18th century, the Age of Theories and Systems.

"We see the great theorists of the time," Garrison writes, "as Emerson has described the gods, each sitting apart in his own sphere 'beckoning up to their thrones,' yet somehow Hippocrates and Sydenham, Vesalius and Harvey, Celsus and Paré, seem nearer and more accessible to moderns than Stahl or Barthez, Bordeu or Boerhaave, Brown or Reil" (13).

In the essay of Dr. Bell, we find a rather poignant complaint on the sterility of the physiology of the period, a physiology aptly described as necrological, in contrast to the physiology developed in the present century which is essentially biological. Dr. Bell wrote:

> That science, physiology, it must be confessed has thus far been of little service to practical medicine—nay more, its values and delusive lights have served rather to mislead, than to guide us from its earliest history to the present era.
>
> The humoral, the chemical, the mechanical, the physico-mechanical systems of physiology, of Cullen, of Brown, of Darwin, of Rush, and shall I say it? of Broussais, are a few of the consequents of the pre-

* Hippocrates thus insisted that "A physician's studies should include a consideration of what is beneficial in a patient's regimen while he is yet in health" (12).

> tended application of the principles of physiology to the healing art. Their physiology was imperfect in part, and in part false; and as a consequence, their doctrines are mere assumptions of unproved, and as time has demonstrated, unprovable facts, or downright imaginations; and just so far as they respectively, have had an influence in turning away the mind from the discovery and consideration of facts, and their application of experience, just so far have they been the cause of incalculable injury to man, and to the progress of science.

Deprived of the robust empiricism of the Hippocratic medicine, and finding the physiology of the period fragmental in knowledge and confused in theory, the physicians of the 18th and 19th centuries found refuge in the then flourishing science of morbid anatomy. This science at least deals with tangibles. To quote Bell again:

> Practical medicine 'must mainly rely for all that is true, and valuable, and capable of being applied, upon the knowledge of pathological anatomy or the changes produced by disease, and upon the internal indications which mark these morbid alterations. The former of these auxiliaries to the healing art is comparatively a subject of modern origin. Not a century has elapsed since the great work of Morgagni on the seats and causes of disease was given to the world, the first valuable contribution of pathological science; after him in slow succession appear the labors of Portal and Baille, of Corvisart and Bichat, followed in more recent times by the bright galaxy of French pathologists, as Boyle, Andral, Laennec, Louis, Cruveilhier, and Hope, Carswell and others in England, whose labors will be felt to the latest days of medicine because they depend upon facts for their eternal basis' (15).

One can see from this how completely physiology and physiological thought were divorced from clinical medicine. That Bell was not alone in his belief may be gathered from the words of Rokitansky who in 1846 wrote, "Pathological anatomy should be the base not only of the knowledge of physicians, but also of their practice as it contains all there is in medicine of positive knowledge" (16). Virchow carried this thought to its extreme in contending that there is no such thing as a sick body that is disordered in all its parts. He maintained that no doctor can systematically think of a morbid process unless he is able to assign it a place in the body.

The phenomenal development of bacteriology strengthened the conception of diseases as specific entities and appeared to justify that type of diagnosis which concerns itself primarily with the morbid process and little, if at all, with the human being involved. This was so very much the case (and still is so today) that von Behring gave it as an article of faith and conviction that all diseases are unique processes caused by unique forces or agents, and that all therapy to be successful, must be directed against the etiological factors. As a corollary, Behring maintained that all efforts directed toward improving the health of the living organism or toward raising its resistance more often lead to havoc than to the desired end.

At this juncture, I should like to illustrate the pervasive and misleading influence which these concepts had upon medicine, by citing a very interesting incident. In 1901, Sir Patrick Manson addressed the Epidemiological Society of London on the Etiology of Beri-Beri. In this address he reviewed and evaluated the then current theories on its cause. Among these he included the theory of Dr. Eijkman of Batavia, and mentioned specially Eijkman's experiments showing that the pericarp of rice, or rice polishings, would both cure and prevent the disease. Manson, however, was not impressed by Eijkman's work. He said:

> To my mind, the theory which conforms best to all the known facts in respect to the etiology and pathology of beri-beri is to the effect that this disease is purely an intoxication produced by a toxin elaborated by a germ whose nidus is located outside the human body; that in this respect beri-beri is on all fours with alcoholism, the germ of which is the yeast plant, the nidus solutions of sugar, the toxin alcohol, and, to complete the parallel, the pathological effect a peripheral neuritis. There is no evidence to show conclusively that beri-beri can pass directly from man to man like the ordinary infectious disease, yet that it is produced by a living germ is certain. . . . (17)

What is significant in this passage is not Manson's failure to appreciate Eijkman's brilliant work, nor his insistence on looking for the germ causation of beri-beri, but rather his failure to associate the peripheral neuritis of alcoholism and the peripheral neuritis of beri-beri as manifestations of one fundamental physiological disorder. Thirty-five years passed before this was achieved and it was possible only because of the renaissance of biological physiology—or, to use more acceptable terminology, by the rise of the science of biochemistry.

This more than any other is the science of the first quarter of our century. Gowland Hopkins, eminently qualified to speak on this score, said:

> As a progressive scientific discipline, it (biochemistry) belongs to the present century. From the experimental physiologists of the last cen-

> tury it obtained a charter, and, from a few pioneers of its own, a promise of success; but for the furtherance of its essential aims that century left it but a small inheritance of facts and methods (18).

From this very same author, we have these most noteworthy observations:

> The biochemist, when he aims at describing living systems in his own language, comes in contact with philosophical thought. Current philosophy is busy in emphasizing the truism that the properties of the Whole do not merely summarize but emerge from the properties of its parts. It is only necessary for the biochemist to remember that his data gain their full significance only when he can relate them with the activities of the organism as a whole (18).

We are much indebted to the biochemists. They have made certainties where heretofore we had little more than premonitions and the faint shadows of reality. Their achievements in the spheres of nutrition and endocrinology are best known. Their labors, however, have brilliantly illumed the entire field of medicine even to its most recondite and obscure corners. Physiology has been enfranchised by biochemistry, and many seemingly unsolvable problems in pathology such as arteriosclerosis, the processes of premature and of so called normal senescence, and those of the malignant growths have been reformulated in the knowledge and thought patterns of biochemistry.

Since diagnosis draws its vitality from all departments of medicine, it is natural to expect that biochemistry should exercise a most profound influence on diagnosis. And such is, indeed, the case, not, be it noted, in the tests which it offers, but rather and precisely where it "comes in contact with philosophical thought" (18).

The prize essays of the Boylston Medical Committee show that the modern practice of diagnosis by means of instrumental precision is little more than one hundred and fifty years old. On the other hand, the function of the diagnosis was subject to a dichotomy of opinion and definition even at the time of Hippocrates. One school of thought focuses its attention on the morbid process and seeks to deal with it as if it were an entity independent of the person affected. The second school is concerned primarily with the person and looks upon disease as an episode in his life processes. While the first group tends to utilize specific curative agents, the second group depends more on the *vis medicatrix naturae*. In the ancient world, and even up to the 17th century, the first school prevailed.

Since then, and until the beginning of the 20th century, the second school, which regards diseases as specific entities, and diagnosis as a telling apart of diseases, has held sway. During the 20th century, there has come into being the science of biochemistry, giving rise to biological physiology, and validating the first, or Hippocratic, version of the function of diagnosis. I will not pass judgments. The castigation of historical periods and personalities is a fatuous sport and I have no intention of setting men or ages in a sort of ascending or descending scale of values. True Hippocratic diagnosis rings more true than does the cellular pathology of Virchow. But Hippocrates lived and functioned in a much simpler world.

We can now recognize that the diagnostic minutiae of the Cnidian practitioners, derived as they were mainly from variable subjective impressions, could not but seem like so much futility to the clear thinking Hippocrates, who was all too well aware that, "Life is short, the Art long, opportunity fleeting, experience treacherous, judgment difficult." On the other hand, the empiricism of Hippocratic medicine, much diluted and much corrupted in its passage down the ages, could not but prove puerile to a world grown complex and inquisitive.

Weary with the thousand years of scholastic garrulousness, the sciences, medicine included, turned to facts, to demonstrable realities. In medicine, the so called seat of morbidity soon came to light. Morgagni found it in the organs, Bichat in the tissues, Virchow in the cells. Because of this, disease came to be thought of as a concrete reality and diagnosis as merely the task of identifying that reality. In the past hundred years, diagnosis, like crime detection, developed very clever instruments and technical procedures wherewith to discover and identify the malefactor. Medicine, however, has grown in other directions as well. The humors of Hippocrates have reappeared in new guise; so has the psyche. In consequence, the seat of disease has acquired a meaning like that of "the seat of government"—namely as the accidental or arbitrary place whence radiate forces that affect the whole economy.

Time and increment of knowledge have made it possible to reconcile the schools of Cos and Cnidus. But, we must confess, they are not entirely reconciled in the present-day practice of diagnosis. While, therefore, we may not find fault with our forefathers, seeing the limitations under which they labored, can we do otherwise than find fault with those of our contemporaries who, in their diagnosis, and perforce in their therapies, still labor within the restrictions of morbid anatomy and of specific etiology, and are unwilling or unable to see the function of diagnosis as essentially the definition of a clinical problem affecting a given individual to be solved therapeutically when possible?

REFERENCES

1. *Library of Practical Medicine.* Boston: Perkins & Marvin, 1836, vol. VII.
2. *Ibid.,* pp. 16-17.
3. BRECHER, A. *Les Etapes Historiques du Diagnostic Médical.* Paris thesis, Paris: Jouve, 1935.
4. BARKER, L. F. The development of the science of diagnosis. Baltimore, 1916.
5. KREHL, L. Ueber der Entstehung der Diagnose (Opus 8). Tubingen: Schnürlen, 1903.
6. HIPPOCRATES (W. H. S. Jones translation). *Ancient Medicine.* New York: Putnam, 1923, Vol. I.
7. *Ibid.,* vol. II, p. x.
8. LITTRÉ, M. *Hippocrates.* Paris: Baillière, 1844, Vol. II.
9. HIPPOCRATES, *op. cit.,* Vol. II, p. xvii.
10. MICHAËLIS, L. S. The limitations of histology. *Lancet,* 1939, 1: p. 186.
11. WHITE, W. A. *The Meaning of Disease.* Baltimore: Williams & Wilkins, 1926.
12. HIPPOCRATES. *Regimen in Acute Diseases,* Book xxviii.
13. GARRISON, F. H. *History of Medicine.* Philadelphia: Saunders, 1929.
14. BELL, L. V. In: *Library of Practical Medicine.* Op. cit.
15. *Ibid.,* pp. 12-13.
16. BROWN, W. W. *Lancet,* 1938, I, 278.
17. MANSON, P. Etiology of beri-beri. *Lancet,* 1901, II, p. 1391.
18. HOPKINS, F. G. *The Problem of Specificity in Biochemical Catalysis.* London: Oxford University Press, 1931.

7

The Epidemic Constitution

Like almost everything which makes life worth living, said Major Greenwood, scientific epidemiology began in Ancient Greece (1). In the books of Hippocrates entitled *Airs, Waters, and Places* and *Epidemics I-III,* we have the beginnings of epidemiology. The first exhorts the physician to appreciate the influence of environment, season, and mode of life, on health and disease. The second offers, in a sense, case notes to illustrate the propositions of the first.

There are critics who find fault with these books, for intermingled with the astute epidemiological observations are to be found comments on critical days, and on concoctions, crisis, and crasis; these they find repugnant. But such critics lose sight of the basic thought. What entitles Hippocrates to be considered the founder of scientific epidemiology is not his speculations on the origin of the Scythians' impotence, nor his theory on the critical days, but rather his understanding, vast and profound. That understanding is of Man's relationship to his universe both immediate and remote. This appreciation is the leaven in all the genuine works of Hippocrates. It is the warrant for his rejection of the supernatural or deistic origin of disease. It illuminates and rationalizes his therapeutic practices. It accounts for his dependence on Nature to effect the cure. Man's susceptibility to the forces in his environment, and their effects on his health are best revealed in Hippocrates' epidemiological books. As Jones, his translator, observes, these are without pretension to literary form but constitute "the most remarkable product of Greek science" (2). In them, Hippocrates advances the simple thought that Man's *private* ills are chiefly the result of his own ignorance and of his slovenliness, but the epidemic diseases are the result of inimical forces, of disequilibria in Man's environment. In *Airs, Waters, and Places* Hippocrates says that he who wishes to pursue properly the science of medicine must consider the effects of seasons and winds, the properties of waters and the soil, and "the mode of life also of the inhabitants that is pleasing to them, whether they are heavy drinkers, taking lunch, and inactive, or athletic, industrious, eating much and drinking little" (3). Even this short passage reveals his insight—a penetrating appreciation of Man's position in the intricate web of Nature.

It is easy and pardonable to read into the writings of Hippocrates more than he ever knew or intended, and to credit him with wisdom and knowledge born in later years. But our evaluation of the writings on epidemic diseases is free of these faults. It would be difficult, rather, to prize them excessively, for they are unique and stand alone for many ages. In what has come down to us from the ancient medical writings, there is nothing that even remotely suggests that in these matters there had been a forerunner to Hippocrates. Nor do any of the speculations of the contemporary philosophers correspond to the basic idea propounded in his writings on epidemiology (4). On the contrary, Hippocrates, in his *Nature of Man,* shows scant respect for these theories and speculations of his contemporaries.

In *Epidemics* we come upon the Greek term *katastasis.* The authoritative translations of Hippocrates render this as "constitution." Liddell and Scott define it as "a state, situation, condition, constitution, quality," and over the years it has acquired other meanings. In the Hippocratic works, however, it connotes environmental factors contributing to the engenderment of epidemic diseases. The importance of these factors was recognized by the two men responsible for reviving epidemiology some thirteen hundred years later—the French physician Gulielmus Ballonius and Thomas Sydenham. Ballonius (1538-1616) carried on the best Hippocratic tradition—to observe, to report, to reflect. In his *Epidemiorum et Ephemeridum,* published posthumously in 1640, he gives the *katastasis* of the years, and then reports the cases he had seen. We have in these works a catalogue of clinical records. But we have little else. Ballonius follows the pattern but adds nothing to the knowledge proferred by Hippocrates. With Sydenham it is quite otherwise. He too returned to Hippocrates, but he went further than Ballonius in pursuing the problems of epidemiology. His epidemiological writings offer us no clinical case records, but they do tease the heart of the matter, the epidemic *katastasis*—or, as Sydenham called it, the epidemic constitution. Sydenham's thoughts on epidemiology have been examined closely by Major Greenwood, from whom I borrow this lucid summation:

> The complete morbid process of an epidemic disease is made up of two parts; the first is specific (the a, b, c, & d., of the formula), subject to secular modification and also to short period oscillations—i.e., it is a doubly periodic function of the time. The second part is generic, common to all species of epidemic diseases and a function of some terrestrial conditions included under the term "Epidemic Constitution" (5).

It is this second part, the generic component of the epidemic constitution which constitutes Sydenham's most valuable contribution to epidemiological thought.

His works on epidemiology gave impetus to the study of the subject; but the later works are lacking in philosophical insight and understanding. They are provincial rather than catholic. They are painstaking and scrupulous collections of meteorological data. They are inspired by the vain hope that the secret of epidemic diseases could be wrested from the collected data on barometric pressures, temperatures, humidities, wind directions and velocities, and rainfall. The two-volume edition of Sydenham's collected works published in Geneva in 1736 includes twenty-one contributions on epidemiology from the pens of twenty authors. These are all devoted to reports on climatic conditions prevailing in given localities during given periods of time, and to notes on the diseases current during those periods and in those locations.

Sydenham was the last of the great English physicians who were nurtured in the ancient medical lore which the Renaissance had resurrected and revivified. With him the Renaissance came to an end and a new age was ushered in—the age of modern science, with its instruments of precision, and its inductive techniques.*

Thought was now on a new tangent. Man found anew his own "bright earth" and, himself. With consuming eagerness he set out to explore the microcosm. With the aid of his balances, his microscopes, his thermometers and barometers, his measuring rods and his chemical retorts he uncovered the wonders of the universe. A new enchantment was upon him, one that alienated him from his former devotions. It is this new enchantment, the limitless faith in inductive science, that accounts for so many men's eager scrutiny of the atmospheres for the secret of the epi-

* Within the lifetime of Sydenham, Harvey published *De Motu Cordis,* Descartes his *Méthode;* Boyle performed his revolutionary physico-mechanical experiments; Malpighi initiated his histological studies; Leuwenhoek discovered the protozoa; Hook published his *Micrographia,* John Graunt drew up his *Bills of Mortality,* and Newton issued his *Principia.*

demic diseases and for the conviction, shared also by numerous others, that the noxious principle could be isolated from the complex of man's physico-chemical environment.

The *katastasis* of Hippocrates was for the while forgotten. But the study of epidemics continued, nay was pursued with even greater intensity. This study developed along three tangents: statistical, historical and bacteriological.

The statistical study was initiated by John Graunt, the son of a London draper, who himself became a prosperous shopkeeper and a Fellow of the Royal Society. In 1662 Graunt published a volume of statistical deductions based on the Bills of Mortality. He thus opened a new terrain which yielded to his followers most illuminating data on the dynamics not only of epidemic diseases but of a vast variety of other social and biological phenomena.

The history of epidemic diseases was always, of course, of continuous interest to Man. Toward the end of the 18th century, however, it was cultivated as a special discipline. Creighton's *History of Epidemics in Britain* is without doubt the *capo lavoro* in this field. It is rich in scholarship, profound in understanding and enormously wealthy in factual data.

Before the influenza pandemic of 1918 swept the earth, most of the historical data was regarded by most epidemiologists and physicians as only so much curious lore, showing the blind gropings of the pre-bacteriological eras. However, the devastating influenza of 1917-18 jolted at least a few among the epidemiologists out of their smug and patronizing state of mind. They rediscovered the precious worth of the historical studies and they have since made splendid use of them.

The last of the three lines of investigation—the bacteriological—is too well and too commonly known to require description. We need only recall that, with the discovery of the disease-producing bacteria, epidemiology promptly became identified with bacteriology. Pettenkofer's was the last brave stand of the "constitutionalists" against the bacteriologists. Thereafter, bacteriology held undisputed mastery over epidemiology. There were, of course, rebels and heretics; but they were as voices in the wilderness. Greenwood neatly sums up:

> It is true that some of the leaders of the victorious bacteriological army, including Koch himself, warned us that the discovery of parasites and the elucidation of their life histories left much of the mechanism of herd illness unexplained, but some of the commissioned officers and all the camp followers of the army would know

> nothing of this caution. It came to be believed, is still believed by a majority, that epidemiology, from the scientific point of view, is a mere appendix of bacteriology, that when the means of infection and the vehicles of infection have been identified, the problem of an outbreak of herd sickness is solved. All the ideas of the ancients were dismissed as archaeological lumber and the work of such writers as Farr, Brownlee, and Ross politely ignored, taken to be mathematical, and therefore intellectually respectable, but of no practical importance (1).

Such was the state of epidemiology during the first decades of the present century. Such it is this very day for most medical men. Two departments share between them the whole terrain of epidemiology—the statistical and the bacteriological. The last two decades, however, have seen a revival of interest in that which has for so long been forgotten and neglected—the *katastasis* of Hippocrates, the epidemic constitution of Sydenham.

The precipitating cause of this revival was the great influenza pandemic; but prodromal signs of disaffection can be noted among a small body of epidemiologists; disaffection with the neat and final assumption that the discovery of the *materies morbi* and of the methods and agents of their transmission resolved all the problems of epidemiology. The influenza pandemic inspired these dissidents with greater courage. Crookshank (6), Greenwood (1), Goodall (7) and Hamer (8) are the names outstanding among those who after 1918 "aroused greatly increased interest in the study of epidemics from the natural history point of view, and tended to discourage meek acceptance by epidemiologists of a belief that all that was required of them was to rewrite epidemiology in terms of causal organisms" (8).

In 1925 Crookshank spoke up in fine sarcasm:

> Whilst leaving the bacteriologists to pursue their researches to a successful issue in the seclusion of their own laboratories—for it were impious to believe that persons who ignore clinical and epidemiological data are not the predestined solvers of clinical and epidemiological problems—it may be profitable to discuss briefly two questions that, although nowadays regarded—at any rate in the best medical circles—as hardly worthy of scientific investigation, have nevertheless engaged attention since the earliest ages. These questions are, first, that of the periodicity of the recurrent pestilence we now call influenza, and secondly, that of the dependence of these recurrences upon, or their correlation with, what used to be called telluric and cosmic influences (9).

The exploration of these two problems, the periodicity of recurrent pestilences, and their dependence or correlation with "what used to be called telluric and cosmic influences," now yields astonishing and illuminating information: astonishing because unanticipated; illuminating because it conforms with our best knowledge in medicine.

In the effort to trace the periodicity of recurrent pestilence, one realizes that history presents a spectacle which can be properly described as "a succession of new plagues for old." This realization invalidates old beliefs, for it has been common to think of historical time in relation to epidemics as divisible into two portions; one enormously long, and the other comparatively short. The line separating these time portions corresponds to the period of the discovery of the pathogenic microorganisms. On one side of the line the epidemic diseases ravaged a helpless mankind, while on the other side modern science mastered, one by one, the plagues of antiquity. But this distinction is misleading and erroneous. History presents an unbroken succession of plagues.

Some of these are as old as mankind. But others are of later origin, and some are very modern indeed. Bearing in mind that we are considering diseases in their *epidemic* form, and not as nosographic entities, we cannot help but recognize some herd diseases to be what the Germans call *Zvilisationsseuche,* plagues of modern civilization. Among such we can list tuberculosis, cholera, typhoid, diptheria, scarlet fever, cholera infantum, and perhaps certain of the psychological disorders, notably schizophrenia. Among the ancient epidemic diseases—those prevalent before the Christian era—we can list bubonic plague, malaria, and typhus, while during the medieval ages we can count smallpox, leprosy, syphilis, and influenza. All of these disease entities have most likely existed since the most ancient days; it is only as epidemic diseases that they are new or recent. Granting that the *contagium vivum* was ever present, why was it that tuberculosis, for example, did not achieve the magnitude of a great epidemic disease until the 18th century? Why was not Europe plagued by cholera, or diphtheria, or typhoid until what we call modern civilization became well advanced?

There are some, of course, who deny the validity of these questions; who maintain that Europe was indeed plagued by these diseases, but that physicians lacking diagnostic and clinical acumen did not recognize them. To this protest the gentle words of Richard Mead form a fitting retort.

> For it must be believed that the first masters of our art who are so careful in describing and distinguishing the signs of all diseases

> would not have briefly mentioned them but would have described them at length if they had but known of these at once terrible and contagious diseases (10).

There can be no doubt that some epidemic diseases have been, and are, new sprung in the succession of time. And their origin is rooted in what used to be called telluric and cosmic influences. Does this last statement sound like a profession of faith in astrology? Then it misleads. Who can gainsay the splendid findings of modern climatology, the painstaking work of Elsworth Huntington and of C. A. Mills, which reveal most definitely the bearing of climate upon the prevalence of disease? By telluric and cosmic influences, however, I intend more than climate, more than even airs, waters, and places. I mean all that was embraced by the Hippocratic *katastasis*—the entire physical environment of the people and in addition their cultural, industrial and economic status.

As a brief and somewhat tentative illustration of the way in which telluric and cosmic influences can help to explain the historical succession of plagues, let us review the experiences of the European peoples, notably the English, during the past three hundred years. This period corresponds to the development of the modern industrial system, which has seen the substitution of the machine for hand tools, the growth of the factory and of the modern industrial community, and the creation of a new social class, the proletariat—the class that has but one commodity to sell, its labor power. Such is the common summation of the technological, economic changes of the Industrial Revolution. But this period also saw other changes, of "telluric and cosmic" character, changes which affected large masses of people. Humanity experienced an unparalleled dislocation in its environmental relationships. Never before had there been such population density, such prolonged and close compaction of persons in factories and slums. The Industrial Revolution removed large masses of people from the soil, distanced them from their food sources, changed their diets, altered their foods, and bound them by an exacting discipline never before experienced. The Industrial Revolution broke up the rural community, disrupted the homestead, dismembered the family. For millions of human beings "airs, waters, and places" were changed, for the worse. The whole social and ethical realm was altered. Old values lost their validity, old relationships their force and strengths. In the light of all this, can we doubt that these "telluric and cosmic influences" engendered an "epidemic constitution," which favored the rise of the *Zivilisationsseuche*? And can we doubt that, in order to overcome these plagues, the *epidemic constitution* must be altered?

This is a belief long shared by the more profound students of epidemiology. Sydenham groped for it, but never seemed to grasp it clearly, though Greenwood believes that he did.

> The bacteriologist—or, at least, his popular exponent—holds that all diseases can be attacked and conquered seriatim by specific measures; isolate the organism, "stamp it out" or procure an artificial immunity and that disease is "conquered." But if my interpretation of Sydenham's constitutions is correct, all that can be achieved in this way is either to reduce the number of stocks upon which a stationary fever may be grafted or to reduce the number of stationary fevers, leaving the stocks upon which the remainder may be grafted untouched. *Naturam expellas furca, tamen usque recurret,* hence Watt's theory of substitution, and Sydenham's constitutions. So the problem of preventive medicine becomes wider and we are led to ask whether what is wrong with the unhealthy may not be not infection with this or that germ but—unhealthiness, even as the chief trouble of the poor is not addiction to public houses but just plain poverty" (5).

The dominant significance of the epidemic constitution was also appreciated to some extent by William Farr, for in his Thirtieth Annual Report he wrote:

> It is, however, by no means proved that the general mortality under unfavourable sanitary conditions is much reduced by rendering a child insusceptible of one type, while he remains exposed to all other types of zymotic disease (11).

Dr. Ozanam, writing in 1817, differentiated clearly between the epidemic proper and the epidemic constitution. He defined the epidemic constitution as "an indeterminate period during which diseases occur, which, though they seem to have different characteristics, nevertheless have the same origin and the same diathesis. It is an unique disorder of which the various forms are, so to say, only symptoms and which requires only one general method of treatment" (12).

Again Ozanam states:

> The epidemic constitution has a more general influence upon the human being, but its effect is felt only in an irregular and diversified manner producing a variety of diseases; whereas the effect of the real

epidemic is more direct, more uniform and more marked and neither hidden nor disguised as that of the former (13).

All of these authors, and others beside, sensed the significance of the epidemic constitution, and defined its nature with varying degrees of acuteness. Most of them conceived of it in terms principally of climatological and terrestrial factors. They knew there was more than these elements in the epidemic constitution, but they did not know the nature of the unknown "more." They could not even conceive of it. They, as all medical men then, thought of noxious states as due to the presence and operation of inimical agents or forces. They could not conceive of morbidity arising from the *absence* of subtle and essential factors.

But then this realization—this recognition of disease resulting from a minus rather than from a plus state—is the most recent achievement of medical science. It is rooted in the epoch-making discoveries in endocrinology and nutrition. This partly accounts for the vain gropings of the epidemiologists of the preceding centuries. They searched Man's realm for a something that was not there, in a manner that could not reveal it. They sought for a positive entity. They contemplated biological Man as the stationary passive fixed entity upon whom the forces of the universe play their mysterious will.

This viewpoint is evident in two remotely diverse authors. Ludwig Edelstein in a philological analysis of the Hippocratic book *Peri Aeron* is distressed by Hippocrates' preoccupations with the healthy man. Edelstein contends that "To be healthy means: not to be ill." The life of the healthy, he believes, does not concern the physician. In this brilliant study Edelstein shares in the reigning beliefs that disease is the positive state, that it is the resultant of aggressive forces which assault Man's constitution, and that health is only the absence of disease.

The other author is von Behring, who states his credo in the following words:

> . . . For we are of the opinion that in combating diseases we can achieve more by attacking the causes of disease than by an attack on the living cells and organs.
>
> Until now we only know that even the best intended, direct attacks on living cells and organs in order to animate or to stimulate them into a state of modified activity, are more likely to harm the cells and organs, than to bestow upon them more health and resistance" (14).

We know today that it is eminently possible to influence the living cell. We know that to a very great extent the competence of the specific disease-producing agents to injure the living body depends upon the telluric and cosmic influences which antecedently affected the living body. The influences are collectively embraced in the epidemic constitution.

By all these considerations, and by their implications, we are compelled to conclude that what Hippocrates intended by *katastasis* is the more important factor in epidemic diseases. Modern medical advances have validated his contentions, and have elaborated on the components of the epidemic constitution.

Insofar as medicine fails to ameliorate the interrelationships of man and his life's realm, it can succeed only in deferring mortality—not in decreasing morbidity. To the extent that mortality is deferred and life prolonged, morbidity multiplies and increases.

REFERENCES

1. Greenwood, M. *Epidemiology: Historical and Experimental.* Baltimore: Johns Hopkins, 1932.
2. Jones, W. H. S. (translator) Hippocrates. New York: Putnam, 1923, Vol. I, p. 141.
3. *Ibid.*, p. 72.
4. Friedrich, C. *Hippocratische Untersuchungen.* Berlin: Weidmannsche, 1899, pp. 130, 162.
5. Greenwood, M. Sydenham as an epidemiologist. *Proc. Roy. Soc. Med.* London: 1919, XII (epidem. sect.), pts. I and II.
6. Crookshank, F. G. (Chadwick Lectures) (Abstr.) *Medical Press,* 1918, clvii, 291, 310, 329.
7. Goodall, E. W. The Epidemic Constitution. *Proc. Roy. Soc. Med.* London: 1927-28, xxi (epidem. sect.) I.
8. Hamer, W. *Epidemiology Old and New.* London: Kegan Paul, 1928.
9. Crookshank, F. G. *Epidemiological Essays.* London: Kegan Paul, 1930.
10. Mead, R. Quoted by J. D. Rolleston in: *The History of the Acute Exanthemata* (Fitzpatrick Lectures). London: Heinemann, 1937.
11. Farr, W. Quoted by M. Greenwood in *Crowd Diseases.* London: Williams & Norgate, 1935.
12. Ozanam, J. A. F. *Histoire Médicale Générale et Particulière des Maladies Épidémiques, Contagieuses et Épizootiques.* Paris: Lyon, 1817, p. 40.
13. *Ibid.*, p. 42.
14. von Behring, E. *Gesammelte Abhandlungen zur ätiologischen Therapi von ansteckenden Krankheiten.* Leipzig: Thieme, 1893, p. lxx.

8

Social Medicine and the Epidemic Constitution

It is not customary nor quite proper to draw the moral before the text is cited; yet I shall do so here. The moral I offer is "when in doubt, turn to history"; my text is "the meaning of Social Medicine."

Any one who has attempted to discover precisely what Social Medicine is and how it may differ from the other divisions of medicine knows how frustrating that quest can be. Each writer on the subject defines Social Medicine according to his own ideas. Stieglitz speaks of it as "Public Health and Preventive Medicine—come of age." John Ryle defines it several times in varying terms. "Social Medicine as we conceive it," he wrote, "is concerned with scientific disciplines and improvements of preventive and remedial practice based thereon, and not with political planning" (1). In his *Changing Disciplines* Ryle writes: "Social Medicine, deriving its inspiration more from the field of clinical experience and seeking always to assist the discovery of a common purpose for the remedial and preventive services, places the emphasis on *man*, and endeavours to study him in and in relation to his environment" (2).

Professor Crew of the University of Edinburgh defines Social Medicine thus: "Social Medicine rooted both in medicine and in sociology includes preventive medicine in this sense as well as industrial medicine, which is surely more than a variant of toxicology, but it differs from these in that it is not merely or mainly concerned with the prevention and elimination of sickness but is concerned also and especially with the study of all social agencies which promote or impair the fullest realization of biologically and socially valuable human capacities. It includes the application to problems of health and disease of sociological concepts and method" (3).

W. Hobson, Professor of Social and Industrial Medicine, Sheffield University, England, describes Social Medicine as an attempt to "link together clinical medicine and preventive medicine in the hope of benefit to both."

George Rosen responds to the question, What is Social Medicine, in the following terms: "Historically, the appearance of a concept of social medicine has occurred in response to problems of disease created by industrialism. To a very considerable extent the history of social medicine is also the history of social policy (welfare). Concerned at first primarily with the new class of industrial workers and their problems, social medicine can today be conceived in a broader sense to include various social groups" (4).

Rene Sand, Professor of Social Medicine at the University of Brussels, writes, "Social Medicine thus comprises: medico-social demography (statistics, polls, surveys); medico-social anthropometry (anatomy, physiology, psychology); medico-social pathology and clinical surgery (etiology, semeiology or diagnostics, nosology, therapeutics in the true sense of the word); social hygiene—here the expression is clearly defined and leaves no doubt (organization, institutions and methods, comprising the medico-social factors relative to health education, prophylaxis, legislation, insurance, distribution of medical services, and social service). Social medicine, the same way as medicine itself, is composed of: anatomy, physiology and psychology—pathology and therapeutics—hygiene" (5).

These quotations show that those who have labored on the problem have a common something in their respective definitions. However, that *something* is neither sharply defined nor really graspable. Furthermore, their differences are more impressive than is their accord. This nebulosity in the definition of Social Medicine has provoked certain souls to opine that it is "a much ado about little" and the sport of those who love to pour old wine into new bottles (6).

Such a cavalier dismissal of the subject however is not allowable, for those who belabor the issue are not only in earnest but count among their number men and women who are outstanding in clinical medicine, in public health, and in epidemiology, and who have put great effort into the advancement of Social Medicine, sometimes at cost to themselves.

In accordance with the injunction "when in doubt turn to history," I pick upon the historical personage who first employed the term Social Medicine—Dr. Jules Guérin (1801-1886), editor of the *Gazette Médicale de Paris.* He gets scant notice in the annals of medical history. Robinson mentions him with some derision, reporting that at the age of 80 he challenged Pasteur to a duel (7). Ackerknecht recalls the more creditable feeding experiments carried out by Guérin in 1838—experiments in which he fed dogs on a diet lacking in calcium and thereby induced rickets (8). Castiglioni mentions Guérin in an inclusive roll call of the men who contributed to the development of orthopedics. For Guérin, beside being an active editor, a prolific medical journalist, a redoubtable advocate of many causes, was also a busy practitioner of orthopedics, to which he contributed many innovations and inventions.

In the year 1848 Guérin was 47 years of age. On February 22 of that year the reign of the Citizen King Louis Philippe came to a quick and inglorious end. The Second Republic followed, and in the *Gazette's* issue of March 3 the lead article is entitled *La République et la Médicine.* In this article Guérin called upon French medicine to guide the French people toward a better life.

> The medical profession is in essence both liberal and republican. The physician by training and experience is conditioned to hate prejudice and to love progress. The intelligent cannot but perceive how medicine bears at many points upon communal, governmental and economic life. Medicine, therefore, better than any other profession can guide the social organism. In public hygiene medicine proffers the sovereign means for the amelioration of the lives of the poor, the workers, and of the entire human race. To attain this there is need for a liberal and progressive government; a widespread knowledge of the true significance of medicine, conceived "from its highest and widest horizon," and the harmonious cooperation of the medical profession.

Guérin felt that the liberal and progressive government was at hand, and that the encompassing influence of medicine upon society would be readily appreciated, but he had some misgivings as to the harmonious cooperation of the profession, whose motto appeared to be *Chacun pour soi et tous contre autrui.*

In the following issue (March 11), he returns to the theme, addressing himself directly to the Corps Médical de France. Here he first employs the phrase Social Medicine. "It is eight days," wrote Guérin, "since we said to our confrères: The republic opens a new era to science and to the profession."

We have already had the occasion to point out the numerous rela-

> tions which exist between medicine and public interest, but these relations, indicated at a time when the social framework was too narrow and too ancient to contain them, could not be conceived of except as the partial applications of a medicine in some respects ideal. But today, when all the barriers of the past drop before progress, this ideal medicine can and must become a reality. The time has come to assemble all of the indecisive and separate activities differently termed medical police, public hygiene and legal medicine, to combine them together and to raise them to a high significance under the more appropriate denomination of Social Medicine.

To illustrate what he intended by Social Medicine, Guérin then asked a host of rhetoric questions.

> To whom better does the resolution of the great problems of the amelioration of the inferior classes belong? Who better than the physician can show the direct way for the development of the moral by the physical, from the education of the children of the poor, to the expurgation of vice? Who better than the physician can determine the usefulness and humanitarian relations between the capacity for work, at different ages, and the requirements of different industries? By whom, if not by the physician will the causes of the physical deterioration of the "working class" be determined . . . and the power of rendering them more healthy, more robust and more happy? A great problem now occupies our minds—increase of wages and reduction of hours of work. This difficulty, examined in the light of Social Medicine, does it not appear subject to an easy and happy solution? Reduction of the hours of work will fatigue the worker less, and increase of wages will increase his energy and his well-being and will permit him to improve and increase his nutrition. The consequence of these two gifts, so affrightening in appearance to industry, will be better and more productive labor. It is simply the case of the horse that runs faster, in less time, for being better fed.

In the following issue of the *Gazette* (March 18), the lead article, appearing under the heading *Social Medicine,* distinguishes between Social Medicine and Socialist Medicine, and says:

> The object of Social Medicine is to indicate all the circumstances in which medicine can aid in the social organization or the welfare and amelioration of society. It does not therefore prejudge any kind of medical theory, philosophical or political. It serves them all without adopting any.

The heading *Social Medicine* at first appeared regularly; but, after a few months, interest seemed to wane and by the end of 1848 it all but disappeared from the columns of the *Gazette*. Furthermore, the subjects treated under this heading were of an odd mixture. Much space was devoted to the question of whether Europeans could become acclimatized to Algeria. Other matters dealt with were the abolition of prison labor, a project for the establishment of mineral water spas for factories, and the bearing of salt marshes on the abolition of the Salt Tax. The editor apparently was not himself too clear as to what subject belonged under what heading. Thus, a contribution by Marc d'Espine on *The Effects of Affluence and of Misery upon Mortality* was printed under the heading *Revue Hygiénique.*

All this suggests that Guérin did not have a well-defined idea of Social Medicine; in fact, he soon turned to other problems. Nevertheless, his venture, slight and brief though it was, is instructive. Clearly his concern with Social Medicine derives not from medicine but rather from a social change—the overthrow of despotism and the inauguration of a liberal régime. "La république ouvre à la science et à la profession une ère nouvelle" (March 11). Now that "toutes les barrières du passé s'abaissent devant le progrès," medicine will and must rise to its high mission.*

Guérin rested the achievement of social medicine upon social reform; this may be why he petered out so soon. For the Revolution of '48 was short lived; by 1850 the reaction was triumphant throughout Europe.

Guérin was not alone in his belief that social reform would open great possibilities for Social Medicine. In Germany he had his counterpart in Rudolf Virchow, who, quite like Guérin, turned journalist and fought "the reaction" in the columns of the weekly *Die Medizinische Reform.*

Virchow and others among his contemporaries are credited by some with having conceived of medicine as "a social science." But this term implies far more than is warranted. Virchow, Guérin, and others saw the social usefulness of medicine, but not medicine as a social science. They urged the public and those in authority to appreciate that *what* medicine knew about the origin and the prevention of disease *could be* and *should be* applied socially, that is by society, for the good of mankind. The burden of their argument was that the knowledge which medicine had acquired was capable of social, as well as individual, utility, or, to phrase it crudely, that the physician could treat a community as well as an individual. I can see in this the application of medical science to social needs and for

* The reader is referred to Ackernecht's excellent review of Hygiene in France, 1815-1848 (9).

social ends. I can *not* see in this the conversion of medicine into a social science.

At this point we may draw some profit from our study of Guérin. It is evident that one possible interpretation of the meaning of Social Medicine is "the application to society, i.e. to the group, or to many groups, of the knowledge which medicine has, bearing on disease prevention, and the promotion of the well being of the social group." This "social application of medical knowledge" differs, of course, from the practice in which the physician treats the individual patient.

Once this possible interpretation of social medicine is appreciated, its correlated opposite naturally comes to mind—namely, the application to the individual, by social means, of such knowledge as medicine may have that bears on the well-being of the *individual.* This too can be taken to be one of the possible interpretations of Social Medicine; of course, the two definitions thus considered are not mutually exclusive. As a matter of historic experience, both have been advanced simultaneously and we may recognize them better when we name them by their more common designations—the first being *public health and preventive medicine,* and the second, *government medicine.*

At this point we appear to have come around the circle to about where we started, and were these two definitions the only ones possible, then Social Medicine would indeed be "a much ado about little" and "the sport of those who love to pour old wine in new bottles." But Social Medicine must mean more than public health, preventive medicine, and government medicine; and indeed there is still another interpretation possible—and the only one I hold valid. Social Medicine is that medicine which envisages the derivation of *both* disease and health from the nature, structure, and operation of the total milieu into which the individual is born, in which he grows and lives, and wherein he reproduces his kind.

Though I've labored to make this definition descriptive, inclusive, and clear, I feel that without an exposition of its historical derivation it must seem more literary than real.

We have seen that the term "Social Medicine" was coined a little over a hundred years ago; and that after a short flare the agitation for it petered out. When and why did it revive? Before trying to answer this question, I must reject the argument that there has always been some interest in Social Medicine, shown by concern with demographic data, industrial hygiene, workmen's compensation, sickness insurance, social work, etc. In actual fact, this motley of interests and agitations has nothing to do with Social Medicine. Again, I cannot agree with Professor Sand when he traces the history of Social Medicine "by digging at its roots, and following them one by one from their origin in remote centuries until they unite into that common trunk which has emerged into view some 40 years ago" (10). One does not clarify the history of Social Medicine by making it coextensive with the history of medicine.

Current interest in Social Medicine has a definable dynamic and a determinable origin. Its dynamic is both suggested and witnessed in the autobiographic note which appears in the preface to Ryle's *Changing Disciplines.*

> I attempted to crystallize some of the ideas born of experience which has come to me since I left London for Cambridge and Cambridge for Oxford, and by degrees transferred my energies from work in the field of clinical and personal medicine to new ventures in the field of social medicine—from studies (in a more academic regard) in individual pathology to studies in social pathology . . .
>
> I have asked myself what was troubling my mind during the period of transition referred to above. Looking back, it has seemed to me that, while Medicine—through scientific and technical advances—has greatly gained in potentiality during the past quarter of a century, it has, in the process, become less surely attuned to some fundamental human needs—to the deeper personal needs of the individual and to the broader social needs of the group or community. In the midst of great social changes we have not succeeded in registering and explaining the accompanying changes in the quantity and quality of many of our main diseases, some of which I shall later refer to as our "modern endemics" (11).

I would in particular underscore this last sentence, for it defines a major part of the dynamic of the revived interest in Social Medicine. Others before Ryle noted this failure "in registering and explaining the accompanying changes in the quantity and quality of many of our main diseases." Indeed, the specific instance in which this failure stood forth in ghoulish prominence was during 1918 and 1919 when influenza swept through most of the world.

That was a shocking experience, the more so because it was entirely unexpected and contrary to what the world, both lay and scientific, had been led to expect. That expectation was advanced by the bacteriologists who on the basis of some impressive though isolated experiences taught that Man had mastered the menace of epidemic diseases. In England in particular, and in the United States to a lesser degree, the influenza pandemic instigated a reassessment of epidemic thought and theory. Crookshank, Hamer, Goodall, and Greenwood were the leaders of this movement in Britain, while Webster of the Rockefeller Institute contributed to it in the United States.

Seen in retrospect, the protest made by these men was rather mild and their challenge negativistic. They insisted that epidemic diseases could not be accounted for in terms of causative organisms alone. "The germ theory," they pointed out, "when it carried everything before it, in the eighties, swept epidemiology off its feet and it was some time before the importance of *soil* (as well as of *seed*) again became fully recognized; even then to allude to the possible influence of a 'tertium quid' was felt to be in bad taste" (12). Crookshank developed the argument a bit further. He urged that the *epidemic constitution,* as conceived by Hippocrates, Ballonius, and Sydenham, should be reconsidered. "One thing at last is clear," he wrote, "if we take heed of the despised 'telluric and cosmic influences' inferred by the older writers and demonstrated by scientific observation in these latter days, we are not thereby under the necessity of dispensing with bacteriological research. Far from it: we may perhaps come to a better understanding of those relations between Man and the microbe that, too often, are expressed in terms of plague and pestilence" (13).

Greenwood contributed to this revival of interest in the epidemic constitution by reviewing and interpreting Sydenham's writings in epidemiology (14).

In this challenge to bacteriological epidemiology that came as an aftermath to the 1918-1919 influenza epidemic, I am persuaded to see the beginning of the current interest in Social Medicine. And the reason for this I would set forth in the terms of etiology. Crookshank, Hamer, and their associates did not add "telluric and cosmic" factors to the known bacteriologic and other noxious agents merely to hypothesize greater burdens to crush suffering mankind. They rather saw them as means to a better understanding of "those relations between Man and the microbe that too often are expressed in terms of plague and pestilence." In this is reflected the core matter of Social Medicine, which looks upon man as a creature symbiotically related to all there is on earth, in it, and in the heavens too.

But in justice to the contributions of their successors, we must not credit these early pioneers with more than is due them. They are distinguished in courage and vision. But still they were too much on the defensive.

They felt obligated to first protest against the presumptions of the bacteriologists, and then to advance their own versions. But in effect they had more to say of the Old than on the New epidemiology. To them the way to progress was by a return to the past. "Indeed," wrote Crookshank, "if we wish truly to progress, we must get back—and the sooner the better—to Hippocrates, whose empirical observations and whose few, yet grandly simple synthetic generalizations and inductions remain, and must ever remain, the foundations of all true Medicine based upon the observation and study of Nature, of Nature's ways, and of Nature's remedies" (15). Hamer devoted a chapter of his book to the Return of the Hippocratic Method.

It was left to the followers of these pioneers—not to return, but to *go forward* with Hippocrates and to apply the Hippocratic method to the study of the new plagues. Ryle refers to them as the modern endemics and gives as an example gastric and duodenal ulcer.

> We have watched these diseases—which were at one time, judging by earlier records of the clinic and the dead-house, relatively rare—becoming in the course of two generations two of the most common of all. Their incidence is still rising. If the combined total of living persons who have or have had an ulcer in America and the British Isles could be computed, they would be found to number, not tens or hundreds of thousands, but millions. Every endeavour, orthodox and unorthodox, medical and surgical, has been made to discover a cure, but with no very outstanding or encouraging results. Animal and laboratory experiments have carried us but a very little way in the assessment of cause. And yet the causes (for ulcer will probably find its place among the "multiple stress" diseases) must have been developing contemporaneously with rising incidence. A disease which was once rare can become so again. Until we study the victims of the disease at first hand and in relation to their work, their total occupational experience, their communities, their food, their habits and anxieties, and their innate predispositions, are we likely to obtain the answer to our question? (16)

It was the mounting awareness of, and the increasing preoccupation with, the so-called modern endemics that in effect engendered the current interest in Social Medicine. This in turn has led to a revival of interest in the Epidemic Constitution.

The modern endemics include a number of disorders which cannot be fitted into the scheme of classical epidemiology. "Multiple stress diseases" are a totally new category in the lists of pathology and involve totally new concepts in etiology. The very term *stress* is difficult to visualize and to fit into our medical vernacular; and *multiple stress* only compounds these difficulties. One can readily demonstrate the noxious effects of tubercle bacilli, diphtheria toxin, smallpox virus, or metallic poisons, but the morbid and noxious effects of *stresses* are a challenge to the imagination.

The "modern endemics" furthermore do not seem to have the familiar socioeconomic distribution. It is not those in the lowest social strata who are most subject to them. The incidence of diabetes, coronary disease, hypertensive disorders, gastric and peptic ulcer, exophthalmic goiter, suicide, and psychiatric disorders such as schizophrenia and manic depressive psychosis does not have the same socioeconomic pattern as the incidence of, say, tuberculosis or infant mortality. Then, too, the morbidities which concern the physician now include divorce, delinquency, infertility, alcoholism, non-criminal social misbehavior, as well as great variety of disturbances in affect function—the so-called psychosomatic disturbances such as colitis, migraine, allergic reactions, sexual frigidity, psychic impotence, and anorexias—and also the disintegrative art patterns and cultisms which are so numerous and widespread today. Out of these awarenesses has issued the suspicion that perhaps society itself is sick. This suspicion comes close to an awareness of the Epidemic Constitution. The concept of a sick society is common in sociology and in economics, but it is entirely new to present-day medicine—though it was known in ancient medicine.

In his excellent work *Psychosocial Medicine: A Study of the Sick Society,* Halliday refers neither to Hippocrates nor to Sydenham, nor does he mention Paracelsus or the term Epidemic Constitution; yet, among all the writers on Social Medicine (he prefers the terms psychosocial medicine, but his theme *is* social medicine) none has come closer to an understanding of the Epidemic Constitution as it bears on Social Medicine. The following thoughts, taken from his book are in the best tradition of Hippocrates and in the spirit of Paracelsus. Speaking of recent changes in the world of the adult, Halliday touches on urbanization and on the increasing separation of man from the outward roots in Mother Earth. We may surmise that urbanization "has increasingly tended to cut off more and more persons from the times and tides of nature which instigate and exercise deep-seated emotional responses." This passage and the one following, bearing on the increasing disregard of cosmic and biological rhythms, would have delighted Theophrastus Bombastus:

> The growing indifference to seasonal and diurnal rhythms and the

> increasing dissociation of the individual from the deepest levels of his emotional life were not solely a function of increasing urbanization but also were influenced by the expansion of the "machine," developments in transport, and the introduction of artificial lighting. The invention and spread of such terms as timetable, day shift and night shift, and piecework illustrate this tendency. The working rhythms peculiar to each individual were increasingly disregarded and socially disapproved (17).

The Paracelsian conception of the Epidemic Constitution is further reflected in Halliday's discussion of the increasing frustration of manipulative creativity; the increasing rapidity of change in the structure of society which has resulted in an obsessive concern with "social security," the increase in standardization and the repression of individual expression, and the increasing absence of aim and direction in life (18). These many and rapid changes in society—in the exploitation of men and women, of the earth (both on its surface and in its depths), and of the atmosphere—have profoundly altered the Epidemic Constitution. In Paracelsian terms, both the macrocosm and the microcosm have in recent times suffered deep and lacerating changes, and the results are strange and painful to behold: They yield us among other afflictions, political and cultural, also the modern endemics.

From all this we can appreciate in what respects our contemporary proponents of Social Medicine "see better and deeper" than did their predecessors. To Crookshank, Hamer, Greenwood, Goodall, and their associates, the "cosmic and telluric" forces were but a *tertium quid*—the third member in a triad of which the first two were "the germ and the host," or "the seed and the soil." But those who today understand the full import of the cosmic and telluric forces, the Epidemic Constitution, know that it is not a *tertium quid* but rather the *prime determinant* which embraces all else. Seed and soil are included in and are themselves affected by the Epidemic Constitution, and in this understanding lies the meaning of Social Medicine. By this understanding one can grasp that unless the Epidemic Constitution itself be altered, the manipulation of seed and soil can yield only partial and temporary results, as when by the aid of antibiotics one saves a sufferer from pneumonia—only to have him shortly thereafter succumb to a cerebral hemorrhage or coronary accident.

It should now be clear wherein Social Medicine differs from preventive and from government medicine and why it cannot be equated to them either by extension or by addition. They are separated by the insurmountable difference in the conceptualization of *etiology*. In preventive medicine and in government medicine, this is rather direct, simple, and also naive. In Social Medicine, on the other hand, it is conceived as being coextensive with, and indeed a function of, the Epidemic Constitution—that is, of "the nature, structure, and operation of the total milieu into which the individual is born, in which he grows and lives, and wherein he reproduces his kind," as I have defined it above.

Etiology as conceived in Social Medicine is complicated and difficult to grasp. This is a serious handicap to the propagation of an understanding of Social Medicine. Yet I know not how this obstacle can be eliminated or circumvented. The idea *is* complicated and it cannot be simplified. All we can hope for is that with experience the medical mind will become accustomed to dealing with multifactored situations and dynamics. I suspect that necessity will provide the experience, and experience the competence. Such is certainly the case in modern physics—where the menacing reality of atomic energy compels us to an understanding of at least quantum theory. In medicine the compulsion is likely to come from just those instances where our prevailing theories fail to account for real events. During the war years England was in mortal fear of an influenza epidemic. The epidemic never occurred—and Lord Horder wrote *The Modern Troglodyte* (19), an excellent essay in the Paracelsian tradition, to explain why.

Many years ago it was forecast by certain epidemiologists and statisticians that the American Negro problem would be "solved" by tuberculosis—or, to put it more bluntly, that the American Negro would be liquidated by *Tbc.* Time and experience proved them wrong. These prognosticators also held that *Tbc.*, as the White Plague, would be totally eliminated among the whites. On this score, too, they were proved wrong. Experience has shown that many of our "etiological assumptions" are wrong. Bad housing is associated with many evils; but good housing does not eliminate all the evils with which bad housing is associated. The elimination of some diseases does not appear to invariably reduce by so much the *total* of morbidity, but rather to shift or to alter morbidity, in character and in time of occurrence. Our mounting burden of chronic disease and disability appears to argue that such is indeed the case.

My original thesis had a double aspect: first, that when in doubt, one should turn to history; and secondly, that Social Medicine can best be understood in terms of the etiological function of the Epidemic Constitution. In the light of medical history, I have attempted to expound what

I deem to be the dynamics of the origin and operative meaning of Social Medicine.

REFERENCES

1. RYLE, J. A. *Irish Journal of Medical Science,* July, 1948, pp. 289-286.
2. RYLE, J. A. *Changing Disciplines.* London: Oxford University Press, 1948, p. 11.
3. CREW, F. A. E. Social medicine: An academic discipline and an instrument of social policy. *The Lancet,* 1944, li, p. 6324.
4. ROSEN, G. What is social medicine? A genetic analysis of the concept. *Bulletin of the History of Medicine,* 1947, xxi, 5, p. 730.
5. SAND, R. *Vers la médicine sociale.* Paris, 1948, p. 580. Transl. from the French.
6. GIBSON, T. *British Medical Journal,* 1949, ii, p. 388.
7. ROBINSON, V. *The Story of Medicine.* New York: 1931, p. 411.
8. ACKERNECHT, E. *Ciba Symposium,* 1944, Vol. 6, p. 1844.
9. ACKERNECHT, E. Hygiene in France, 1815-1848. *Bulletin of the History of Medicine,* 1948, xxii, pp. 117-155.
10. SAND, R. What is social medicine? *Acta Medicinae Legalis et Socialis,* 1948, No. 1.
11. RYLE, J. A. *Op. cit.,* (Ref. 2), pp. v, vi.
12. HAMER, W. *Epidemiology Old and New.* London: Kegan Paul, 1928, p. 2.
13. CROOKSHANK, F. G. *Epidemiological Essays.* London: Kegan Paul, 1930, p. 55.
14. GREENWOOD, M. Sydenham as an epidemiologist. *Proc. Roy. Soc. Med.,* 1918-19, xii, (Epid. Sec.), pp. 55, 61.
15. CROOKSHANK, *Op. cit.,* p. 20.
16. RYLE, J. A. *Op. cit.* (Ref. 2), p. 20.
17. HALLIDAY, J. L. *Psychosocial Medicine: A Study of the Sick Society.* New York: Norton, 1948, pp. 121, 122.
18. *Ibid.,* p. 121.
19. HORDER, T. In: *Journal of the Royal Society of Arts,* 1941, Vol. 89.

9

The Birth and Death of Specialties

> *I am convinced that the conception of specialism dominant today is a wrong one, and that helpful as this specialism has been in many ways, nevertheless, instead of enlightening, it tends to darken understanding in a cloud of detail. That each new phenomenon discovered by methods simple or recondite is of importance in adding to our knowledge of disease, is accepted as a truism, and on that ground specialism seems justified. But there are other matters in the recognition of a phenomenon beyond its discovery which are essential to the progress of medicine.*
>
> SIR JAMES MACKENZIE (1)

It is interesting that, while much has been written on the rise of specialties, no one, to the best of my knowledge, has noted the fact that specialties also die. Nor has much study been given to the generic phenomenon of specialism in medicine—that is, to the varieties of determining forces which engender it in medicine. There are a number of competent histories, each of which treats of the origin and development of an individual specialty. But there is no history of specialism as such (2).

Surely it must have struck many a thoughtful person that the phenomenon of specialization, not merely in terms of the specialties developed but as a dynamic experience within medicine itself, merits study and exposition. How is it then that there are so many individual histories of individual specialties but no analytic or dynamic history of specialism?

While this is an intriguing problem, the answer, in effect, is quite simple. Most medical historians identify the history of specialism with the history of modern medicine. Castiglioni (3), for example, dates the origins of specialism from the 17th century. "Thus," he writes, "at the end of this (the 17th) century, when the cooperation of medicine and the natural sciences was being emphasized, we already see outlines of the essential features of the great structure of experimental science. Already various specialties began to be detached from the main trunk. . . . Here we have an extensive preparation for modern medicine."

Castiglioni's vision of modern medicine as a continuous and accelerated detachment of various specialties from the main trunk of medical practice is shared almost universally; indeed medical history seems to support and validate this vision. And yet, persuasive as this vision may appear to be, there crowd on one's mind a number of troubling awarenesses and a host of questions that somehow cannot be reconciled with it.

There comes to mind, for example, the history of surgery. In the days of Hippocrates, the physician was also a surgeon and he was no less esteemed in the one role than he was in the other. Some among the followers of Aesculapius were notably skilled in setting broken bones, in lancing festering sores, and in dressing the wounds caused by sword and spear, and they were properly noted for their skills. But they were physicians first and surgeons incidentally.

The Hippocratic books on surgery (*On Wounds and Ulcers, On Hemorrhoids, On Fistulae, On Injuries of the Head, On Fractures, On Reductions of Dislocation*) were addressed to the very same practitioner who found instruction in the Aphorisms and who was taught to see the ecologic relations of Man in *On Airs, Waters, and Places.* Surgery was a phase of medicine, even as were diet and pharmacology.

It is reported that the Romans did not hold the physician in high esteem. But insofar as the Romans did prize the physician, they favored him equally as surgeon. With the decline of Rome and the advent of what is so picturesquely, but erroneously, termed the Dark Ages, surgery somehow became separated from medicine, and thereafter its practitioners were looked upon as a "scurvy lot." Physicians then were no longer surgeons, and surgeons were not physicians. They were, in the main, barbers or butchers by trade, or otherwise itinerant handymen. Yet the Middle Ages were not without some truly famed surgeons: Guido Lanfranchi (d. 1315), Henri de Mondeville (1260-1320), and Guy de Chauliac (1300-1367), to name but three. It is noteworthy that these men who did so much to advance surgery are as one in lamenting the decline of the practice of surgery by physicians. "Physicians regarded it as undignified to practice surgery, and especially blood letting, but left them both in the hands of barbers," complained Bruno de Longoburgo in his *Chirurgia Magna.*

What had happened to bring surgery down to so low a level? And what afterwards redeemed it and made it not only an honored but, as I am told, a highly rewarding practice? Surgery, it should be noted, was rehabilitated long before the advent of modern medicine—that is, before bacteriology, asepsis, and anesthesia. Of John Hunter (1728-1793) it was said that "He found surgery a mere mechanical art, and left it a beautiful science," and also that he "made gentlemen out of surgeons." The latter statement, if taken literally, is a dubious compliment, but the observation is intended to be taken historically rather than literally. I raise these questions with no intention to pursue them. My purpose in citing the history of surgery was merely to point out that the vision of the development of medicine as a process whereby the specialties detach themselves from the main trunk to flourish thereafter is just not correct. It does not conform to reality.

Nor for that matter is this vision supported by the history of other specialties. It may not prove flattering to the "professional origins" of the orthopedist, the dentist, the oculist, the proctologist, the urologist, and the dermatologist, to name but a few, but it is true that the practitioners in each of these specialties from the Middle Ages down to the recent times were in the main minstrels, mountebanks, and quacks—that is, sharpers of every kind and variety. I am not sure we are entirely fair to these stalwart pioneers, for sharp they surely were, and they had to be; no doubt among them there were also many men of high skill, fine dexterity, and of much practical, if not academic, wisdom. Be that as it may, the lithotomist, the bone setter, the lens coucher, the fistula mender, and the extractionist were specialists who plied their specialties long before medicine itself had become diversified.

We must conclude, then, that specialization is not concomitant with, nor is in itself a gauge of, the advancement of medicine. Historically, medicine was never more specialized than as it was practiced in ancient Egypt. In *The Persian Wars* (volume ii, p. 84), Herodotus reported that in Egypt "Each physician applies himself to one disease only, and not more. All places abound in physicians; some physicians are for the eyes, others for the head, others for the teeth, others for the intestines, and others for internal disorders."

From this we may conclude that in the history of medicine specialism is a problem apart. It is not, as some have affirmed, and many believe, the inevitable concomitant and the logical resultant of scientific progress.

Indeed, the long view of the history of science reveals the pattern of periodic diversifications in interest and knowledge—that is, of specialization—followed by periods wherein the synthetic unification of knowledge is achieved. Science is never more innately consonant and rewarding than during its unitary stages.

But if specialism is a problem apart, then what indeed is it? Before treating of it further, we require precise definitions of specialism, specialties, and specialists. For on examination we find that the term and the concept of a specialty and of a specialist relates to a number of diverse professional functions. There are specialists in single diseases, as for example, the tuberculosis specialist, or the syphilologist. There are specialists in the use of singular instrumentalities, as, for example, the x-ray specialist. There are operational specialists, as for example, the surgeons and the obstetricians. There are specialists in single organs, as the eye specialist, and of single systems, as the neurologist or the gynecologist. It is true that none of these specialties is insular and the specialists who pursue them have an overlapping knowledge of other departments of medicine. Yet the significant conclusion that can be drawn from the most ample catalogue of the different references which the terms specialty and specialist carry amounts to this: The common factor in medical specialism can only be described in negative terms. A specialist is one who does not practice comprehensive medicine. He exercises his skills only in some subdivision or in some partial function within the larger framework of medicine.

This definition is not intended to be, nor is it, basically derogatory. It is purely descriptive. It is also historically most suggestive and most significant. Let me project two of its telling implications. One is that with the advance of medicine comprehensive medicine as such cannot be practiced. The other telling implication is that the summation of the practices of the specialties in effect constitutes the practice of comprehensive medicine—that is, of total medicine. Here we encounter the reversal of the famous dictum that the whole is greater than the sum of its parts. Specialism implies that "the sum of the parts is equal to the whole." Group practice does not publicly subscribe to these convictions, but they are inherent in the rationale and procedures of group practice, which, in effect, amounts to the deliberate structuring of "basic specialists" in a close cluster pattern.

Specialism in medicine, however, long antedated group practice. Group practice is merely the latterday logical development of the theoretical concepts on which modern medicine is founded. These theoretical concepts can best be described as specificism in the etiology of disease and in therapy. The concern of modern medicine was deliberately and avowedly fixed on disease. The specific causes of specific diseases, the specific treatment of specific diseases, and the specific prevention of specific diseases comprise the three principal branches of modern medicine. The pursuit of these concerns is best effected by specialization. Hence our specialists and specialties, all of which, with the possible and partial exceptions of pediatrics and obstetrics, are concerned and occupied with disease.

Modern medicine has not been concerned with health, save only in the negative sense of "the seeming absence of disease." It has been almost entirely occupied with the "conquest of disease." It has openly subscribed to the faith that health is to be gained only in the conquest of disease. Von Behring formulated, professed, and proclaimed this faith. It has not been disavowed, at least not by an appreciable number of medical leaders, though some few, the late John Ryle for one, have protested and have argued that the seeming absence of disease cannot be equated to health, nor is health to be gained in the "serial" conquest of disease.

The concept embraced in the conquest of disease appears very simple. In effect, however, it is enormously complicated and, incidentally, of dubious validity. In its simple and popular form—popular among physicians no less than among the informed laity—it corresponds to Ehrlich's analogy of the magic bullet, which, like the guided missile of the military, finds its mark, the malignant agent, and destroys it. Then there is no more disease, and by that token, the person who was ill is now well. He is healthy.

The interesting thing is that medicine can boast of few specifics, that is, of few magic bullets, and even those deemed to be specifics do not function quite like guided missiles. It is also very questionable whether medicine has conquered any appreciable number of diseases. We may claim that much for medicine only if we embrace under the term medicine all the biological sciences, including the sciences of hygiene and sanitation. But that is a loose, and to my mind not only unwarranted but confusing, extension of the range of medicine. I would limit the meaning of "medicine" to that which is practiced by the physician in relation to his patient. It is, after all, here that we find the specialism with which we are concerned.

In this purview it can be seen that the physiologists have contributed more to the conquest of disease than have the clinicians—that is the medical practitioners, specialists included. Furthermore and perforce, the physiologists have been more deeply concerned with the normal than with pathology. Their contributions have obviated disease by pointing the ways to the maintenance and fostering of health. The physiologists have not been specificists, for health is not a specific factor but the resultant of many contributing correlated factors (witness Claude Bernard's magnificent concept of homeostasis).

I cannot undertake to support this affirmation with many data, nor do I think it necessary that I do so. Yet I would refer to the contributions which the science of nutrition, primarily and essentially a physiological discipline, has made to the conquest of disease, chiefly in enabling us knowingly to promote well-being. One needs but think of the conquest of rickets, with its multiform complications ranging from long-bone deformity and pelvic distortion to tetany, to gain some idea of the protean beneficial effects of this science. Endocrinology is another physiological discipline with far-reaching effects in the conquest of disease. It is worth noting that there is more than a casual relationship between nutrition and endocrine function, as may be witnessed, for example, in the role of iodine in thyroid function. Indeed, it is not all a bizarre assumption that what are classed as trace elements among the chemical components of the body may play a very determining role in the functions of the endocrine system. Our growing knowledge of the operations in the human economy of the trace elements, I am certain, will not only enable us to promote well-being but may contribute phenomenally to the conquest of disease.

On a par with the physiologists in their telling contributions to the conquest of disease stand the public health scientists. Yet their functions, their operations in the field of health promotion and disease control and prevention, are difficult to define. That is so, in part, because their operations are so varied and so numerous and also because, inevitably, some phases of public health have been tinged with specificist theories and ideas. Public health has, like medicine, suffered from an excessive preoccupation with disease. That, however, has been so only during the past hundred and fifty years. During its long history, which extends over more than two thousand years, public health has been, in essence, the science of Man's ecology. Public health, from the most ancient times on, has served and guided Man in the effective manipulation of his environment. This science above all others has enabled man so greatly to increase in numbers and to spread to the four corners of the earth.

The Hippocratic classic *On Airs, Waters, and Places* was a primer in human ecology. I emphasize human, for it lies in the nature of Man not merely to desire salubrious environments but even more to render those places where he lives fitting to his wants and needs. Man is a manipulator and, in a measure, the master of his environment. Animals go to the water hole, but Man sinks wells, builds aqueducts, and in various other ways fetches water to serve his needs—precisely where his needs are. Man, to reiterate, does not helplessly yield to his environment: he manipulates it, he bends it to his will in a thousand ways and more. Of course, the extent to which Man can manipulate his environment with safety, and to his enduring advantages, has its limits. That, incidentally, is a realization not yet fully or widely appreciated. Impressed with the many things man can do and has done with and to his physical environment, many are unmindful of the collateral effects and labor in the persuasion that man can do anything and everything—in time. In this Man is an ecologic ignoramus.

That public health is essentially the science of human ecology is not a common persuasion. I expect it will become so in time. For basically it is a sound and an illuminating identification. Considered in this light, the main enterprise of public health, as well as its major achievements, become intelligible as a consistent performance. Otherwise they seem but a miscellany of separate acts, to be catalogued in such categories as water supervision, sewage and garbage disposal, food inspection, and nuisance control. Even so seemingly singular an achievement as the production of an effective vaccine against poliomyelitis, when examined in its larger and deeper relations, can be recognized as an achievement in ecologic control and adaptation. Commonly it is viewed as a "miracle" in viral immunology. In its lesser dimensions, it is all of that, but in effect it is an ecologic adaptation of great significance.

Since this is a point in the larger argument which we are pursuing, I must develop it in more ample dimensions and in finer detail. Ecology is not a term that can be defined with facility, for it refers not to a thing nor to many things but rather to relations—that is, to relations between things and to the relation of relations between things, the things being of many orders and varieties. As a science, ecology is the study and exposition of the multiple, and often of the subtle, effects which both living and nonliving entities exercise one on another, and the many among themselves.

As far as Man is concerned, ecology is a humbling and a leveling science. It reveals that in the embracing scheme of things, in the scales of ecologic nature, Man weighs no more ponderously than does the vibrio of cholera, the spirochete of syphilis, or the bacillus of phthisis. Contrary to the illusions bred by the evolutionism of the 19th century, Man is not Nature's darling, nor is he Creation's favorite. Ecologic Nature has no favorites and manifestly does not fend for man against the rest of its creatures. Ecologic Nature is seemingly committed to but one objective, to the maintenance of what might be termed a cosmic homeostasis, that is, not to allow, or better still, to disenable, one from among its many kinds of creatures to gain an unbalancing dominance over the rest. When the hawks outbreed the mice and rats, they evoke the ecologic countereffect of starvation—till balance is once again established between hawks and rodents.

That ecologic Nature is not always effective in maintaining cosmic homeostasis, in the rather crude sense, is evident by the historic emergence of certain new species and the disappearance of certain old ones. Man's achieved preponderance, numerically and power-wise, in the living world likewise witnesses the fact that ecologic nature is manipulable. But this is only so under given conditions.

Man is the only one of Nature's creatures who has learned how to deliberately manipulate ecologic Nature. He is not, however, always mindful of the fact that she is only manipulable but never to be corrupted or traduced save with dire consequences. Under any circumstances there is always a premium to be paid, a tribute to be rendered to ecologic nature for every novelty that is introduced into the established order.

Man runs into the menace, or into the brunt, of disaster whenever he forgets this exaction of an ecologic quid pro quo. It is not possible, as was attempted during the Industrial Revolution, to herd great masses of humans into filthy slums, to work them long and hard, to feed them miserably on an inadequate diet, without suffering the retribution of plagues and of untimely deaths. It is not possible, as we are beginning to perceive, to disrupt the traditional and long-established patterns of the familial interrelations of husband and wife, and of parents and children, without encountering the untoward and manifold effects of social delinquency, adult no less than juvenile. The point, of course, is not that we should have avoided the Industrial Revolution with its emergent urbanism, nor is it that we should seek to retain the family pattern of say, the Victorian Era. That is not the point at all. It is rather that we need be mindful of the broad ecologic changes effected by the immediate alterations in the patterns of our existence and seek to compensate for them. That is what public health has endeavored to achieve, whenever public health has been at its best. It is an ecologic compensation to fortify bread with the very elements initially extracted from the grain during the milling process, when the process is an ecologic requisite to the feeding of urban populations dependent for their daily bread on commercial, mass bakers. It is an ecologic manipulation to expose an individual by means of vaccines or other antigens to a controlled encounter with noxious agents in order to achieve deliberately what ecologic nature might accomplish indifferently, to wit, the basis for a coexistence between "germ and man" favorable to the inoculated individual.

Ecology as a science and public health as the science of human ecology are major subjects by virtue of their innate significance and dimensions. I have brought them into my exposition in order to identify them, together with physiological medicine, as the two disciplines which, far more than clinical medicine, have contributed to the "conquest" of disease and to the advancement of well-being—that is, of health. And, as I am sure you must anticipate, it is my conviction that the future in medicine belongs to these two—to ecologic medicine and to physiological medicine, the latter dealing with the normal and optimal internal milieu of the individual, and the former with Man's external milieu, in its broadest and deepest implications.

Yet what of the specialties? Seemingly we have wandered far from our committed theme, but the long excursion was necessary. For I have argued that the specialties were developed chiefly as a result of modern medicine's predominant concern with disease. Then, as we have seen, diseases have been conquered not by the clinical or surgical specialties but by ecologic and physiological medicine. The conquest of certain diseases has effected the death of certain specialties. In this dictum, both "conquest" and "death" must be understood in a relative rather than in an absolute sense.

I have referred to a number of diseases once common and now rare. Among them are rickets, chlorosis, and cretinism. To these we may add a number of other diseases not perhaps entirely rare but certainly of markedly diminished prevalence and of lowered demographic significance. Tuberculosis is one, and an ecologic disease par excellence. Syphilis and gonorrhea assuredly have been conquered in the effective if not in the absolute sense. What then has happened to the veneral disease specialist and to his specialty? The surgery necessitated by the sequelae of the Neisserian infections, in both male and female, but especially in the female, has been greatly reduced. Reflect on what has happened to the surgical otologist whose *raison d'être* were the chronic ear infections and the mastoid involvements? The dermatologist, one of the earliest among the specialists, has perhaps proportionately lost more terrain than any other specialist. Consider, for example, that broad class of skin disorders, formerly falling within the realm of the dermatologist, which have literally evancesced under the impact of the physiological illuminations of nutrition and endocrinology.

With all this in mind, I submit that what has happened during the past quarter of a century is more than likely to be extended and intensified during the coming decades. We have witnessed only the infancy of physiological medicine and the full import of ecologic medicine remains yet to be grasped, even by those in the vanguard of medical progress. Many more specialties will be revolutionized in the not too remote future.

It is not at all playing the vainglorious role of the prophet to prognosticate the proximate resolution of a substantial number of the mysteries that surround certain among the leading causes of death—specifically, of malignant growths, atherosclerosis, coronary disease, and malignant hypertension. To the list I might add, just to come closer to home, the diseases of dental decay. Nor is it too wild a guess that much of the illumination that will dissipate the mysteries surrounding these diseases will come by way of physiological explorations into the normal. To envisage the effects of these much to be hoped for developments, think what a blessing to mankind, and how ruinous for dentists it would be, were it really possible to prevent dental caries. I do believe this possibility will eventuate. I do not, however, think it will be ruinous for dentists. They will simply work more effectively in other directions. Similarly, think how much of surgery will be obviated when we have learned to control the neoplastic growths; this, too, is within realistic prospects.

The combined research attack, now being focused on atherosclerosis and coronary disease, notably along the tangents of the metabolic fate of fats, promises, I am confident, some fundamental insight into the physiological derivation of these disorders. Since metabolism is under the sway of the endocrine system, it is not rash to anticipate the uncovering of some implicated endocrinologic fault in the atherosclerotic processes. Nor should we overlook the apparently significant role of exercise in the retardation of these disorders, as has been so clearly demonstrated in the epidemiologic studies of J. N. Morris.

On the future of cancer research I dare not venture a prognostication, save in the most general terms, namely that cancer, or better the neoplasms, will yield their mystery to physiological research centered on the complexities of embryologic growth, reparative tissue growths, and the mechanisms of their provocation and arrest. Here the morbid and malignant lie too close to the "life creative and normal" not to be under the sway of similar if not identical principles.

It is not my intention to say precisely how these major diseases will be eliminated but rather that they will be in the forseeable future, most probably because of our growth in physiological knowledge and by the cultivation of better ecologic medicine. When that happens, we will witness the "death" of other specialties currently preeminent.

What I mean to convey is this: The future of medical service is not to be envisaged as a continued refinement, as well as increase, in the specialties, with the consequent parceling out of the patient to a host of men, who will care for him and treat his illnesses. I think rather that within two generations medicine as a science, and medical service perforce, will have undergone a revolutionary change, in many respects as profound as that effected by the rise of bacteriological sciences. This revolution will not be brought about by the economic, legislative, or social manipulations of well-meaning men, but by the maturation of those knowledges and intelligences embraced in physiological, and in ecologic, medicine. Unless global disaster puts an end to civilization and to science, the eventuations I have sketched are to my mind inevitable.

I am conscious that I have been somewhat light in my treatment of present-day medicine, including its specialists. I may have thus given an erroneous idea of the esteem in which I hold contemporary medical science and its practitioners. I deem them both of the highest order. Were I grievously sick and had I the choice to be sick in any age in history, from the time of Hippocrates to the present, I would choose none but the present. For at no time in the history of Man has the practitioner of the healing art been as tutored in the skills and as well armed with as great a multitude of means to fend against the ravages of sickness, and even more against pain and suffering, as he is today.

But as I have argued and as is clear to all thinking men, the treatment of disease is not the equivalent of the promotion of health and well-being —and specialists treat disease.

I am not so sanguine in my hopes for mankind, nor so naive, as to believe that man will ever so manage his life as to have no need for "cures" and for the specialist who ministers them. I can envisage an attrition in specialties and specialists but not their total elimination from the medical scene or corps. It is only that I can see the future of medicine as lying in directions other than greater and ever greater specialism.

REFERENCES

1. MacKenzie, J. *Future of Medicine*. London: Frowde, 1919.
2. Rosen, G. *Specialization of Medicine with Particular Reference to Ophthalmology*. New York: Froben Press, 1944.
3. Castiglioni, A. *History of Medicine* (translated and edited by E. B. Krumbhaar). New York: Knopf, 1947.

10

Historical Epochs in Medical Education

Medical historians have concerned themselves primarily with the development of medical science. Relatively little attention has been paid to medical practice, and even less to the teaching of medicine.

There is, in fact, a wealth of information on both teaching and practice, but it is widely scattered. A good deal of it is in the voluminous biographical and autobiographical literature; but this affords only crude and uncritical data. Another and in some respects superior source is the institutional histories of universities, hospitals, and medical schools. A splendid miscellany can be found in the writings of Charles H. Haskins, Lynn Thorndike, Stephen d'Irsay, and other mediaevalists and historians. There is, then, no dearth of material for a definitive history of the teaching of medicine, and yet, with but one or two exceptions, the subject has been dealt with only coincidentally. I am, of course, cognizant of Pushmann's excellent work on Medical Education, but I cannot set him entirely apart; he, no less than the others, wrote under the sway of a persuasion which I intend to challenge.

This persuasion is that historically the practice and the teaching of medicine are direct derivatives of the science of medicine. As the one progressed, so did the others. From the mainspring of scientific insight and knowledge there cascaded a stream of influence which shaped and determined the teaching of medicine and, secondarily, its practice.

One may say: "Well, isn't that really the case? Haven't we seen, these past few decades, how much new developments in the science of medicine have reshaped both the teaching and practice of medicine?"

I would agree that they have. I would also point out that not all recent developments in the science of medicine, psychiatry and nutrition, for example, have been adequately incorporated in the medical curriculum. There is, it would appear, a bias operative in the election of *which* new developments will be accented in the changed curriculum. But, more pointedly, I would argue that what we have experienced, intensively, during the last thirty years, and less sensibly and urgently during the past two hundred, is not representative of the larger historical experience. We are, in effect, passing through a singular epoch in the history of medical education—an epoch in which medicine is dominated by the laboratory, rather than by the sick bed.

I suggest that the history of medical education is divisible into distinctive epochs—and also that medical education is *not* a derivative of the *science* of medicine but rather mirrors the biases, the particular interests, and the preoccupations of those who teach medicine.

In this perspective it is to be seen that the teachers not only shape medical education but also bias the direction in which the science of medicine is pursued. This no doubt explains, in part at least, why the medical innovators, especially when their innovations fall outside the domains of the established schools, or challenge some of their cherished tenets—Paracelsus, Harvey, Semmelweis, Pasteur, Pettenkofer, Freud—encounter so much hostility and opposition. If, then, the teachers of medicine—and, in terms of the present I intend the formal staffs of the medical schools—do wield so much power, then it behooves the statesmen in medicine (whoever they may be) to be mindful of who is privileged to teach and of the criteria by which they are selected.

Stated briefly, my thesis is that the history of medical education is not mirrored in the history of the science of medicine; that medical education has its own and singular history; that this history is divisible into distinctive epochs; and that the characteristics and dynamics of a given period in medical education deeply influence contemporary practice and affect the direction in which the science of medicine is likely to progress. Here I shall restrict myself to a delineation of some distinctive epochs.

That medicine is as old as mankind seems a warranted assumption. "Disease in some form," wrote William Caudill, "is one of the fundamental vital problems facing every society, and every known society has developed methods for coping with disease and thus created a medicine" (1). Man came into being as a social animal. He experienced and was cognizant of injury and disease. Among the earliest of men there were no doubt some individuals, older, more acute and astute, observant and venturesome, who served their fellow men in the ways of a prototype physician. Who taught this early physician? How did he gain his education? His school and his master were one and the same—to wit, experience. For a long time there was no other school.

Among the numerous cave paintings, rock gravings, and sculptures that have been discovered and studied, none pictures or suggests a medical scene. And this is not surprising, for only when Man reached the stage of agriculture did the circumstances of his existence favor the cumulative growth of a transmissible medical culture.

The development of agriculture and the domestication of animals involved the immobilization of the population and the building of permanent homes and shelters. Time and energy were set free for exploring the possibilities of Nature. Discoveries and inventions of far-reaching importance such as metallurgy, pottery and, above all, writing followed soon after the first adoption of agricultural life. Social and religious changes also followed. Fertility rites now formed the chief basis of religion. The scattered groups of independent food gatherers were thus firmly bound together under the authority of a *priest-king*. It is seemingly from the institution of priest-king that the *shaman* derives. But of him, more later.

One significant effect of the development of agriculture was the phenomenal increase in human population. This resulted in a tremendous acceleration of cultural development. Enrichment of culture, Linton points out, depends primarily upon above average minds. These are mutants of unpredictable appearance whose abilities are rarely inherited, and who count no more than possibly one in 3,000 of the population (2). It is more than likely that not a few of the mutants turned their superior intelligence to the practice of healing: hence the shaman. Shaman designates both priest and medical man.

We know little of the Neolithic shaman, but we meet his counterpart in primitive cultures. In paleolithic culture, before the discovery of agriculture, the most important person in the community and the nearest approach to a chief was a shaman. His functions, however, were only sporadic and incidental. Anthropologists commonly attribute to the shaman "hysterical tendencies"; though they do not say what they mean thereby, the characterization is astute and most likely correct.

The medicine man was rarely, if ever, a genuine psychotic. To be a successful practitioner required a firm grasp of reality and superior intelligence. Nor was the average medicine man a charlatan. He believed in his own powers and frequently possessed abilities in what is now called extrasensory perception. He was also, in most cases, an excellent psychotherapist and possessed a knowledge of genuine and non-magical remedies for common ailments. "There can be no doubt," Linton concludes, "that a study of African materia-medica and healing practices would contribute significantly to our own medical knowledge" (3).

During the long period of primitive medicine, the role of healer was open to all. Only the exceptional, it would appear, attained empowering recognition, but the aspiration was free to every man. It was no folly of the Babylonians that they exposed their sick at the marketplace, soliciting those who knew ought of the ailment to counsel with them. For the marketplace, the fair and the cities that neighbored them attracted the venturesome and the informed as well as the pretenders. At first experience was the sole teacher. But with the accumulation of material wealth and the growth of cities, with the division of labor, the development of specialization, and particularly after the invention of writing, rites, mysteries, and esoteric lore were formulated into a *gnosis* and *technê* of medicine that could be passed on from master to novitiate. The teaching of medicine was done by those willing masters to whom the acceptable pupils applied. The teaching of medicine was seemingly as unrestrained as was the pursuit of the aspiration to learn.

Noteworthy, then, are these distinguishing characteristics of the epoch in medical education which has its undefined beginnings in prehistoric times and its end with the rise and growth of the universities: that access to the study and practice of medicine was relatively free, as was also the teaching of medicine. Whosoever chose could learn and teach. There were no schools in the physical sense, though there were "sacred" places and temples. The so-called schools were those of thought, theory, and practice. They were like the invisible colleges of the 17th century, and indeed like the nascent universities of the 1300s. Also they were mobile. Wherever the adherents gathered—there was the school.

It would be easy, but not very relevant, to cite instances which do not strictly correspond to my generalizations—say the Babylonian and the Egyptian. But these were unique civilizations that had run their course before our own historic development took form. And their singular histories, notably that of Egypt, mirror the same patterns of progression which characterize our own experiences. In time, the practice of medicine became professionalized, access to it restricted, teaching the prerogative of an elect, and instruction rigidly formalized. Commenting on the latter stages of Egyptian medicine, Sigerist notes the dominance of the priests and affirms: "Wherever there is a numerous clergy that has a firm grip on the people, magico-religious medicine flourishes at the expense of rational medicine" (4). It appears as if this were the inevitable case, save only that with each succeeding age the priests serve different gods, magic and miracles are of a different order, and what is deemed rational is unique and novel.

I signal the 13th century as the end of the first epoch in the history of medical education because it is then we perceive the beginnings of the restrictive regulations which were henceforth imposed upon the student, the practitioner, and the teacher of medicine.

These restrictive regulations were formulated by the temporal kings and enforced by their temporal powers. Roger, King of Sicily, in 1140, and Frederick II, in 1224, promulgated stringent laws regulating the study, the teaching, and the practice of medicine. "Frederick's edict," writes Garrison, "did much to elevate the status of the respectable physician and correspondingly to diminish the number of quacks" (5). Frederick II thus emerges as the defender of the respectable physician. But he who comes as the defender oft remains as the captor. Henceforth the study of medicine and the teaching of medicine are sheared of a goodly portion of their historic freedom. The "defender of the respectable" ordained that "none of the Salernitan teachers could teach medicine or surgery anywhere but at Salerno, nor any but those duly certified by the King's officers could claim the title of medical teacher. The punishment of death was imposed on the officials who violated their duties in giving effect to these laws" (6).

Similar restrictions were imposed on the students. Envious of Bologna, Frederick II established by decree the Studium, i.e., the University of Naples, as ill fated as it was miserably conceived, and once again with the same restrictions on masters and students as those imposed on Salerno. D'Irsay comments on this eventuation as follows: "This grievous precedent, eagerly imitated at the end of the Middle Ages, marks the University of Naples as the first in a long line of State Institutions, destined to appear everywhere two hundred years later" (7).

Haskins neatly sums up the emergent relations of kings, courts, and universities, in his account of Frederick II: "It is characteristic of Frederick's strongly personal policy that the intellectual life of his kingdom centres in his court rather than in universities, and that the southern universities in his reign show little vigor of life and leadership. His absolute and paternal ideas of government left no place for independent corporations of masters and students living the free and turbulent life of the northern *studia*. So Salerno, which had grown to eminence as a school of medicine without the aid of prince or Pope, found itself tied down by royal statute in 1231 as part of a comprehensive regulation of the practice of medicine, surgery, and pharmacy throughout the kingdom of Sicily, issued in the interests of bureaucratic administration rather than of university development. The course of study is laid down by law, and royal officers are to be present at the examinations. A similar bureaucratic purpose runs through the statutes establishing the University of Naples in 1224 and reforming it in 1234 and 1239. Frederick needed trained public servants, and he preferred to have them brought up in his own kingdom rather than in Bologna and other Guelfic cities of the North" (8).

Many Universities were founded during the 13th and 14th centuries, not all of them, however, by the temporal rulers, for the Church was not unmindful of the potentialities of the universities—for its own ends. The Church had need of clerks, ecclesiastical functionaries, and doctors in theology, no less than the formative states had need for notaries, lawyers, and civil administrators, i.e., literate personnel for its growing bureaucracy. In the race for ecclesiastical prestige and personnel on one side and for power and civil servants on the other, medicine was perforce but little fostered in the universities. Of the two preeminent universities, Bologna was the fountainhead of jurisprudence and Paris that of theology. Padua and Montpellier were the main centers of medical education. Other universities included schools of medicine in their academic ambience, but they were in the main feeble and futile: They had few students and fewer professors.

The teaching of medicine declined grievously. Only the study of anatomy and surgery prospered. Medicine was taught from the texts of Hippocrates, Galen, and the later compilers. The universities provided no practical training, only theoretical indoctrination. It is no exaggeration, then, to say that during this second epoch of our review the teaching of medicine had sunk to a base level, thus meriting all of the opprobrious criticisms directed at it by Petrarch and Paracelsus.

This second epoch calls for some delimitation. To my mind it extends from the 13th to the 17th century. In the latter period we can perceive the emergence of a new era, the beginnings of a new epoch, one that derives from the development of humanism and of inductive science. Both of these developments took place largely outside of the universities, and were in a measure opposed by them. Once again free men joined freely to pursue in common their interests in learning and science. They formed their Invisible Societies (1645), their Academies (1657), their

Royal Societies (1662), and bound the world of the learned in a reticulum of correspondence and reports.

The teaching of medicine revived, and in time it prospered, but the center of its influence was no longer the university lecture hall, but rather the hospital ward. Initiated by Montanus at Padua in 1543, the bedside teaching of medicine was brought to a high degree of skill by Boerhaave of Leiden, whom the great Haller called "the common teacher of all Europe." This epoch is well named "the era of great teachers." Its preeminent men were not infrequently successful practitioners, much favored teachers, and the writers of numerous texts.

The 18th century gave us the great theorists—Stahl, Bordeu, Boerhaave, Brown, Reil, and the other system makers. Garrison finds little merit in them; but, cut free from the bonds of Hippocrates, Galen, and the Arabists, they sought to reconstruct medicine in the patterns of their immediate experience and the contemplation thereof. There was more freedom in the pursuits of medicine—in its study, practice, and teaching—than during the preceding or succeeding epochs.

Here I shall indulge in a brief aside. Medical historians often lament the decline in the practice of medicine during the period extending from the 16th to the very middle of the 19th century. They despair of the blood-letting and purging, of the unbridled use of emetics, and of the therapeutic and pharmacological jungle in which the physician wandered as one both deluded and blind. That the practice of medicine was indeed in a degraded state cannot be denied. But it is, I submit, the historian's obligation to understand rather than to blame. And this period is not difficult to comprehend. It is a transition period, one in which the old was discarded and the new not yet brought into being. Men do not attain to knowledge or wisdom in a single leap. They grope for it, and groping they often wander far from the mark. Were all the theorists and system makers fatuous and futile? Were they not rather earnest men grappling with the unknown? And how many among those we celebrate as the true scientists derived their inspiration, be it only negatively, from those before them who had made the wrong guess, or put forward an erroneous theory? I am inclined rather to regard this period as heroic in spirit, even if modest in accomplishments.

Be that as it may, this third epoch yielded to our own. The beginnings of this are difficult to date (let us say in the 1840s), but its outstanding characteristics are easily discernible. Ours is the epoch of the laboratory and the specialist. "The teaching of medicine as a science," wrote Garrison, "as something of larger scope than its practice, began with the foundation of laboratories and with the gradual assemblage of specialties as units in university instruction" (9). But of these developments Theodor Billroth, writing in 1876, had a rather dismal view: "the object of our modern endeavor is to make the physician's skill independent of tradition, and by means of written records to conserve the art of healing for all time, so that it may be independent of the talent of the individual and may be reduced to an absolute science. All knowledge and skill are to be determined and controlled by means of the laws of arithmetic and logic in order to make everything absolute and permanent." Further he adds: "I doubt if this good will ever be reached, at least in the art of healing" (10).

Some believe that the goal *has* been reached! Certain it is that the dominance of the laboratories and of the specialties has profoundly affected the teaching of medicine. Paradoxical though it may seem, they have displaced the clinician as teacher. In many a medical school the Professor of Medicine is not one schooled and experienced in the treatment of the sick, but rather is noted for his research in the physical or biological sciences. Also, access to the study of medicine has become increasingly restricted. Both the pre-medical and the medical curricula are exacting and quite rigid. The teaching of medicine has become professionalized. To a large extent teaching medicine has become *the* career of "the full time man." What effects all of this has had on medicine, in its embracive and ultimate gauge—i.e. on the life and well being of the people—troubles a good many thoughtful persons.

In conclusion, I submit that medical education has its own, singular history. This is distinct from the history of the science of medicine. Those who teach medicine deeply influence its practice and bias the direction in which its science develops. The history of the teaching of medicine deserves and requires more attention.

REFERENCES

1. CAUDILL, W. *Anthropology Today.* Chicago: University of Chicago Press, 1953, p. 772.
2. LINTON, R. *The Tree of Culture.* New York: Knopf, 1955, p. 86.
3. *Ibid.*, p. 430.
4. SIGERIST, H. E. *A History of Medicine.* New York: Oxford University Press, 1951, vol. i, p. 268.
5. GARRISON, F. H. *History of Medicine,* 3rd ed. Philadelphia: Saunders, 1921, p. 165.
6. PUSCHMANN, T. *Geschichte des medicinischen Unterrichts.* Leipzig: Veit, 1889, p. 176.
7. D'IRSAY, S. *Histoire des universités françaises et étrangères des origines a nos jours.* Paris: A. Picard, vol. 1, 1933, pp. 134-135: "Ce fâcheux précédent, imité avec

empressment à la fin de Moyen Age, désignait nettement l'Université de Naples comme établissement d'État, le premier d'une longue lingnée, qui devait se multiplier surtout deux cents ans plus tard."

8. HASKINS, C. H. *Studies in the History of Mediaeval Science.* Cambridge: Harvard University Press, 1924, p. 250.
9. GARRISON, *op. cit.,* p. 776.
10. BILLROTH, T. *The Medical Sciences in the German Universities.* New York: Macmillan, 1924, p. 2.

11

Humanism and Public Health

My theme embraces both humanism and public health. But humanism is my favorite. In this essay, it bears the same proportion to public health as the horsemeat did in that famous French sausage said to be made 50-50 horsemeat and rabbit—that is, one horse to one rabbit. There is, however, some good warrant for my partiality, for public health is better known and more widely discussed than humanism. Indeed, there is little understanding of what humanism is, so that whoever ventures to discuss it must begin by advancing a definition.

In attempting this, one is confronted by a confusion of assigned meanings. To some, humanism is no more than a nostalgia for the ancient days that comes upon high-school teachers of Latin and college professors of Greek who find their classes dwindling to the vanishing point. Others think of humanism as an historical episode, like the struggle between the Guelf and the Ghibeline—as something that once happened and remains entombed in the chronicles. To still others, humanism means a partiality to the ancient tongues, the badge of an educated person, the show of acquaintance with the wise saws and clichés of the antique authors.

The better schooled may have penetrated the meaning of humanism more deeply. They recognize in historical humanism an episode of capital importance to the human race. They fathom the significance of the revival of Man's interest in Man, the shifting of Man's concern from the remote heavens to the microcosm, Man himself. But even so, humanism remains, even to these, an enthusiasm for the antique—for that which, though present, is complete and passed, like the rare art of the Byzantine mosaic.

Which definition should one accept, even if only as a nucleus for one's own version? In considering this, we can do no better than to begin with the traditional facts, with historical humanism.

The events of that age, so aptly called the Renaissance, are common knowledge. From the sparks engendered in Petrarch's love of Hellenism, there came the flaming enthusiasm of the Cinquecento humanists. Tutored in the school of the ancient authors, these humanists, now grown to manhood, spoke forth in the spirit of the old, but in tongues new and of things contemporaneous.

But here the question must arise: What have they in common? Too many of them seem to cancel each other in their lives and works, so very different are they in respect to personality, character, and even scholarship. And yet, as Taylor observes, "among themselves they formed a band, not of brothers, often of hateful foes, but still of men united in their enthusiasm and pursuits" (1). It is their enthusiasm, their pursuits, that we may hope to reduce to some common denominator of humanism.

The answer to the question, *What were their enthusiasms and their pursuits?* is all too often given with fatal facility. Their enthusiasm was for Cicero, Plato, Aristotle, Lucretius, Pliny! Alas! This answer neither shows nor affords understanding. It is based on bare facts, bare of sense and insight. It is founded on what every history book tells: the awakened interest in antiquity, the search for manuscripts, etc., etc. In all this there is no illumination as to why? or wherefore? In Italy, the ancient cultures —the Roman especially—were never completely lost. In Sicily, Greek was neither a forgotten nor a strange language. The ancient manuscripts were there to be found. All this being so, we are obliged to inquire not only as to the nature of the humanists' enthusiasms and pursuits, but also as to the reasons therefor.

Humanism was not spontaneously engendered; it was not of parthenogenetic origin. It has its genitors—the preceding centuries, those of the Mediaeval Age.

As if responsive to some deep urge, dumbly sensed and little understood, those who write of the Renaissance commence their story invariably with Dante. Dante, however, is not of the *Renasscimento,* nor was he a humanist. Dante was a great Mediaevalist. Yet he does indeed belong to the story of the Renaissance, for his Divine Comedy is both the tomb and the Column cochlis of the Age, celebrating, but also memorializing, the agonies and miseries of Mediaevalism.

In the *Inferno* and *Purgatory,* Dante sums up his passionate and bitter indictment of Mediaeval man, the Church and the monarchies. The vile corruptions of the human spirit and of the institutions are here portrayed episodically with the staccato brilliance of lightning. It was the experienced despairs of the living man that stirred his genius. Better than the host of chroniclers, bogged in the minutiae of their retainers' doings, does Dante portray for us the living, throbbing, anguished Age in which he lived.

This Dantean world is the proscenium of the humanists. This was the world they knew and experienced. Renaissance humanism was a reaction to the frustration and despair that engulfed the Dantean universe. To the humanists, humanism was a *vita nuova,* a new faith, the promise of salvation; *and it can best be understood as a reaction to what Gilbert Murray has aptly called "the loss of nerve."*

From time to time, the human race appears to experience profound moral crises. Its social, economic, and ethical framework then reveals itself to be defective; the mechanisms by which everyday life is transacted prove unworkable. The norms and values by which Man has grown accustomed to measure the worth of things become invalid.

In the reactions of mankind to such crises three patterns are manifest, exemplified in Savonarola, Machiavelli, and Leon Batista Alberti. The first is that of the spirit completely overwhelmed, that, like Savonarola, cries out the vanity of all human life, sets all hope in the hereafter, and makes Death the great liberator. The second is that of Machiavelli, the high priest of Caesarism. The spirit that aches and troubles, the questioning conscience, that child's naïveté which survives in the sensitive man despite years and experience—these are discarded and rejected, and Man is set forth without feeling or faith as an engine of purposeful effort devoted to the achievement of an end wholly encompassed in the individual.

The third pattern is that of humanism. It is the pattern of faith in Man, of hope in Man, of charity toward Man. Though the heavens appear to whirl, the humanist knows that the stars move in their appointed patterns. Neither blind to nor overwhelmed by the temporal disaster, the faith of the humanist and his hope sustain him. As one who has gone astray but is not lost, the humanist retraces his steps to find the familiar landmarks, wherefrom he may set out again, this time aright.

It is thus we need to understand the humanist's enthusiastic study of the ancient classics. For where could he find a faith in Man more native to his own than among the Greek and Roman authors, who lived and wrote when the world was young? The humanists loved not Plato because he was Plato, but because he told of his master Socrates, whose passion for truth and whose faith in Man's competence to gain truth and beauty and wisdom were boundless. It is conceivable that, had any other ancient people or any other literature offered what they found alone in the

Greeks and the Romans, the humanists would have been as much devoted to these as they were to the Greek and Roman authors. But they found no such equivalents; nor have we, since.

The humanism of the Cinquecento needs then to be understood, not as an historical episode, singular or unique, but as an instance in which a reactive pattern possessed by some portion of mankind became prominently manifest in a time of great social duress. Humanism is thus seen to be a pattern for dealing with life's problems and situations, as much and as deeply rooted in Man as are his reactive patterns of "fight or flight."

There were humanists before *the humanists,* and many after them. St. Francis was a humanist. So too were Abelard and Roger Bacon. Later there were Erasmus, Montaigne, Voltaire, Goethe, Anatole France, Georg Brandes, to name a very few at random. All these were humanists, sharing faith in Man, hope in Man, and charity toward Man.

It seems to me, then, that by venturing this far into history, we have acquired the basis for a definition of humanism. Humanism is a way of life. As such it is courageous, hopeful, wise. It eschews alike the doleful perspective of the Vale of Tears and the rude and brutal view that presents the earth as an arena in which all the victories go to the crafty, the amoral, and the strong.

The humanist finds abject renunciation a fatal paralysis of the spirit, and Caesarism the impetuous tantrum of the uneducated intelligence. Neither Savonarola nor Machiavelli is to the humanist's liking, though he understands them both. The distinguishing characteristics of the humanist, and by the same token of humanism, are: large perspectives, willingness to wait for results, competence to endure, intelligence to reconcile divergences, and profound faith in the educability of Man.

The humanist is no Pangloss; he knows that this is far from the best of all possible worlds. He has no illusion about Man either; he sees him as he is, but that vision does not blind him to Man's potentialities. The humanist is an individualist, but with a keen social conscience. The romanticism of the idealist-anarchist the humanist finds puerile, but more repugnant to his soul is that social philosophy which idealizes the pattern of the beehive and the ant hill.

The humanist is neither an anchorite nor a stylite. He is seldom found on the ramparts or the barricades, for, being essentially a teacher, he finds these unsuited to his labors. But to survive is not the main devotion of his life. Humanists have died on the cross; have drained the hemlock cup; have endured exile, poverty, abuse, derision, and neglect. In this larger sense, then, we may speak of humanism as a way for living life, individually and in the aggregate.

Scanning the horizon of history, we can perceive that while each generation had its distinguished humanists, humanism as a dominant ideal prevailed in but few of its sectors. In the Periclean Age, in the time of Cicero, in the gloaming years of Marcus Aurelius, humanism animated and inspired some varying portion of mankind and influenced the destinies of the mass. But with the advent of the Dark Ages, the light of humanism was all but blotted out. For that, it was the more brilliant when it shone forth again in the Renaissance. The development of the new science, however, soon overshadowed the humanism of the Renaissance, and in a fashion discredited it. For that which was old—and humanism cannot be completely dissociated from the ancient literature—was unacceptable to the new science. *De omnibus dubitandum* was the motto of the new school founded by Galileo, Bacon, and Descartes. And yet, humanism was not completely eliminated until the so-called immutable laws of science came to dominate our thinking with a tyranny as complete and exacting as that of the theocracy of Mediaevalism.

In recent years, humanism has again been engaging the interests of men—because the so-called immutable laws of science are seen to be the products of the "thinking patterns" of the human brain, rather than the objective codification of Nature's own injunctions. But the mechanistic philosophy of modern science has been ably examined by Alan Gregg (2); and I must now turn to the other half of my theme—public health.

Modern public health must be distinguished from the hygiene and sanitation of the ancient days. It is as much the creation of recent civilization as is the factory system, and the relation between the two is causal and organic.

The modern public health movement was initiated during one of the late historical periods in which humanism was in the ascendancy. It is rooted in the humanism of the 18th century. The social efflorescence of humanism, as has already been witnessed, is a sure sign that the people are beset by misery. At other times, humanism is a private, not a social devotion. The 18th century was, for the greater masses of mankind, an age of great privation and suffering. It was a century also of great paradoxes. It was the Century of Enlightenment, and also that of absolute despotism.

The humanism of the 18th century, like that of the Renaissance, was rather murky, since its current carried the sludge of many contributory streams. Mixed with the humanitarianisms of the enlightened despot were the primitive sentimentality and romanticism of Rousseau and the atheistic distemper of the materialist philosophers.

In the great public health movement that took place in the second half of the 18th century, Johann Peter Frank is an outstanding figure (3). His *System einer vollstäandigen medicinischen Polizei* is one of the classics of public health. Indeed, the beginning of the modern public health movement is commonly dated from the publication of this masterwork; and there is, in a measure, good warrant for this. As August Hirsch observes, "Until the end of the Eighteenth Century, all efforts to perfect hygiene were made from fragmented and individualist viewpoints. There was wanting a unification of the whole problem, and this Peter Frank achieved in his *System of Medical Police* (3).

That great work was essentially an academic achievement, and had no direct or immediate effect on contemporary public health. But it was the first enunciation of that school of thought which bases public health administration on legal injunction and police enforcement. In this regard, Frank's viewpoint was closer to that of the benevolent despot than to that of the humanist (4). What really matters, however, is not whether public health regulations are codified and carry punitive provisions, but whether they have popular sanction. It is one thing for a law to be desired by and acceptable to the people, but quite another to have it imposed without reference to their wishes.

In the Germanic countries, public health developed quite along the lines of Frank's prospectus, and, since many of our own public health leaders of the last century came under the influence of the German school, this is also largely true of our own public health. It still operates too much in the spirit of the policeman. But the modern public health movement developed first not in Germany but in England, and its character there was essentially humanistic. Sir George Newman wrote: "The story of the evolution in England of the present Public Health Service was not of course isolated. It was the development of a century. It took colour from the changing times and the ever-changing succession of party governments. Its character was derived from the ideas of statesmen and doctors, inspired by an opportunist policy and the growing knowledge of Preventive Medicine. Its trend was, however, directed by two much wider influences, namely, the expansion and interpretation of *Humanism* and an everextending *Education* of the people as a whole."

The modern public health movement, at least in the Anglo-Saxon realm, arose as a movement of protest against the degrading conditions in which a large portion of mankind was compelled to live in consequence of the Industrial Revolution and the growth of modern capitalist economy.

The plight of the English proletariat even at the beginning of the 19th century was horrible. Those degrading conditions have been ably described and documented by Friedrich Engels and J. L. and Barbara Hammond. The Utopians, the economists, and the social philosophers attempted in their respective ways to analyze and to interpret the forces that brought about the New Civilization with all its attendant evils. They advocated a variety of remedial schemes, and by their discussions and agitations they fixed the attention of the governing powers upon the cankerous conditions that afflicted the poor.

It was the revision of the Poor Laws that initiated in England the events which ultimately led to the development of the modern public health movement. In 1832 Lord Grey's government established a Commission of Inquiry into the operation of the existing Poor Laws in England and Wales. Edwin Chadwick, the father of the modern public health movement, was appointed one of the assistant commissioners to the Inquiry. The complete report of the Commission was published on February 20, 1834. In retrospect, it appears nothing less than logical that inquiry should have gone from the administration of Poor Laws to the causes of poverty. It is not surprising then that in 1839, after the presentation of reports by Drs. Neil Arnott, James Phillips, and Southwood Smith on "the prevalence of certain physical causes of fever" and on "physical causes of sickness and mortality to which the poor are exposed, and which are capable of removal by sanitary regulations," a commission was appointed to study the sanitary conditions of the laboring classes of Great Britain. The report of this commission, written entirely by Chadwick, was rendered in 1842. The two reports—on the Administration of Poor Laws and on the Sanitary Condition of the Labouring Classes—had a determining influence on the development of public health. They altered its character, changing it from a humanitarian to a humanist movement. Instead of being moved by a charitable compassion for the suffering masses, it became animated by the conviction that "Man could, by getting at first principles and by arriving at causes which affect health, mould life altogether into its natural cast, and beat what had hitherto been accepted as fate, by getting behind fate itself and suppressing the forces which led up to it at their prime source."

These "first principles" and "causes which affect health" were sought for and studied in the *total* environment of the individual. The total personality (to use a phrase now so very popular) in all its relationships was at its beginnings the concern of the public health movement.

It is incorrect to designate the pioneering public health workers as "sanitarians" unless sanitation be made to mean more than it commonly does. True, the public health pioneers were interested in sanitary improvements, but they were also interested in working conditions, in wages, in intemperance, in illiteracy, in child labor, in crime prevention. Theirs was a broad humanist understanding of the forces that affect health. We find this well reflected in an address by Chadwick, delivered in 1860 before the National Association for the Promotion of Social Science (7). The thesis of his address was that it behooves all communities "to take measure to arrest the unsanitary conditions, which annually slaughter full two hundred thousand persons by preventable disease" (p. 17). The course which he proposes "is, first, to arrest the great infantile slaughter from preventable causes in towns; and next to improve the physical and thence the moral training of all children, especially the children of the labouring class" (p. 10). He goes on to describe the oppressing conditions under which the labouring man is compelled to live —and adds the comment, the wonder is "that the moral, as well as physical combustion is not greater and entirely destructive of the effects of all religious and moral education whatsoever" (p. 15). This is said in the conviction that unsanitary conditions result in moral as well as physical deterioration (p. 20). Chadwick also recognizes the greatest obstacle in the way of amelioration to be "the interest-begotten prejudice and obstinate pessimism which utterly disregards the proved means of prevention and alleges that the 'poor must be poor' as if to be poor it was necessary to be miserable; which adopts as a maxim of ineffable official wisdom, 'never to act until it is obliged, and then to do as little as it can' for the relief of human misery, and recklessly frustrates any attempt to that end" (p. 23).

In this discourse we see reflected the breadth of wisdom and the broad encompassment of public health in its initial stages. All of Man, in all his associations, was the concern of public health. Disease was not charged to the morbific effect of one factor in the individual's environment. It was considered rather to be the resultant of a multitude of factors, and the public health was dedicated to the ferreting out and removal of all the disease producing factors, be they noxious working conditions, long work hours, inadequate wages, bad housing, contaminated food and water, ignorance, or illiteracy. Such at least was Chadwick's devotion, shared by a few of his disciples.

Such, too, were the convictions and devotions of his American counterpart Lemuel Shattuck, though in a somewhat restricted way, for the two were men of different mettle, Chadwick being more of the radical reformer than was Shattuck. In England, Chadwick was relieved of his official functions by the dissolution of the Board of Health in 1854. In the United States, the development of the public health movement, launched by the labors of Lemuel Shattuck, was retarded by the Civil War. However, neither in England nor in the United States did the public health movement suffer a serious setback. In England, at least, it went ahead at an even pace, under the leadership of Sir John Simon, who in 1855 became the central medical officer to the General Board of Health.

In the last quarter of the last century, the development of public health was greatly accelerated by the growth of bacteriology. During this time, however, it lost its humanistic qualities. It became microbistic. Public health shed its concern with working conditions, hours, wages, literacy, and child labor—with Man's total environment. Its preoccupation was almost exclusively with germs, vaccines, serums, fumigation, sterilzation, and quarantine. In all of this, it followed, of course, in the footsteps of medicine. The new public health leaders were medical men. They were not sociologists, economists or philosophers. They were trained in the laboratories, schooled in the newly developed bacteriological Institutes of Europe. Theirs was a distinctly different and a new school of thought in medicine. It goes by the label of Etiological. It is a school dedicated to the conviction that disease—notably infectious and communicable disease—is due to specific causes which, science prospering, will undoubtedly prove amenable to control by specific therapies.

The etiological school of thought was, in its early days, strenuously opposed and vigorously challenged by the humanist partisans.

The history of that conflict is instructive. The outstanding antagonists were Virchow and von Behring. Virchow, in the best of humanist traditions, made social reform the core and vital power of public health. To von Behring, the champion of the etiological school, public health was summed up in the widespread application of the findings of bacteriology. Virchow's public health credo was "full and unrestricted democracy." His public health formula was "education with her daughters Freedom and Prosperity." Von Behring's faith and credo were "sterilization, immunization, and blood serum therapy."

The etiological school prevailed. The practical achievements of sterilization, immunization, and blood serum therapy were great and ever present; and to people who wanted immediate results, the entire philosophy of the etiological school was incontrovertible. It was accepted, not only as itself, but also as a refutation of the humanist viewpoint. Public health thus suffered a narrowing of its field of vision, a shriveling of sympathies, an alienation of its human affinities, and in consequence a loss in its social effectiveness.

To those raised in worshipful awe and admiration of "bacteriological public health" these observations must sound heretical. But they are founded on the facts of history, not on prejudice. Sins of omission can do as much harm as those of commission, and such are the sins, the deficiencies of bacteriological public health.

Much of the glory of present-day public health streams from its artful grappling with the disease problems created by modern civilization. The contest is interesting; but insofar as many of the deeper, fundamental factors—those with which the humanist is concerned—are not affected, the issue of the contest cannot be affected either. The problems are too often solved only "for the time being"; the final issue is deferred. It is not, of course, possible for medicine or public health to solve problems involving social, economic, and cultural factors not under their direct control. But neither medicine nor public health appears to be aware of its limitations in performance and understanding. Each is part of the society in which it functions; and perhaps we should not expect it to be humanistic in a non-humanistic period. Nevertheless, we can and should expect the spirit and the faith of humanism to be urged upon society by the leaders in medicine and in public health. For who is better trained, and better placed to appreciate and to prize humanism?

Nor is this expectation vain. In the past, physicians were prominent among the humanists, and today too we can observe a quickening of the spirit of humanism in some few men in medicine and in public health. This spirit needs nurture, devotion, and appreciation.

REFERENCES

1. Taylor, H. O. *Thoughts and Expression in the Sixteenth Century.* New York: Macmillan, 1920, vol. 1.
2. Gregg, A. Humanism and science. In: *The March of Medicine.* New York: Columbia University Press, 1941.
3. Hirsch, A. *Über die historische Entwicklung der öffentlichen Gesundheitspflege.* Berlin: Lange, 1889.
4. Schmitz, K. E. F. "Die Bedeutung Johann Peter Franks für die Entwicklung der sozialen Hygiene." Veröffentlichungen aus dem Gebiete der Medizinalverwaltung. Berlin: Schoetz, 1917.
5. Richardson, B. W. *The Health of Nations,* p. 27.

12

Doctor and Patient in History

In the passage of time, certain items of medical practice have acquired the status of fundamental principles, the neglect or subversion of which, it is thought, degrades the practice of medicine and radically reduces its effectiveness. Among such "fundamentals" are: "free choice," "fee for service," "the exclusion of all parties intervening between patient and physician," and "the unbreachable confidential nature of patient-physician relations." There are other mythic beliefs about the physician, his privileged position in society, and the uniqueness of his relations with his patients; but the four I have cited are in spirit representative of the rest.

These components of medical practice are commonly regarded as innate in medicine, and, hence, as no more subject to challenge or modification than would be the moral principle "honesty is the best policy." They are propounded as self-evident. And in principle they do, indeed, appear to be desirable, democratic, and dignified, in the sense that they place doctor and patient in the conjunction of free agents, each acting according to his own best interest and judgment. Nevertheless, in *historical experience* they are not the *sine qua non* of good medicine.

Historically the patterns of medical practice have been as varied as conceivably possible. Save perhaps for the basic moral commitments not to willfully injure and not to betray confidences, every condition of medical practice has at some time in history been represented by its obverse. That is most certainly true of free choice, fee for service, the third party in the patient-doctor relation, and the confidentiality of the physician's findings.

Except those derived from the technological achievements of modern times, every form of medical practice is to be found in the historic past.

Thus, in the days of Hippocrates we find the salaried physician who was required to treat the sick without a fee. Herodotus reports (iii, 131) that Demokedes (6th cenutry B.C.) was the community physician in Aegina, receiving as the annual emolument of his office one talent. In Athens, where he served in like capacity, he was paid 100 minen. Later he was called by Polykrates to Samos, and here his annual stipend was 2 talents (1).

Theodor Puschmann describes the *demosieountes* or people's doctors, chosen by the people to serve them in their community (2).

Military medical practice was well defined. Among Xenophon's 10,000, there were eight military physicians. Alexander the Macedonian was accompanied on his military expeditions by four of the most distinguished of the contemporary physicians, Phillippos of Akarnania, Kallisthenes of Olynthia, Glaukias and Alexippos (3).

Rome more than Greece favored the practice of the "retained-physician," i.e., the physician who served the wealthy patrician as "medical famulus." He was usually well paid, but his social position was not one of high esteem. The Roman aristocracy cultivated a dilettante interest in medicine (e.g., Celsus), but it considered medical practice suited only for those of lower extraction, and for slaves. The better known physicians reaped rich rewards; Galen received a fee of 400 gold pieces from the Consul Boethus for medical services rendered his wife. But as Galen observed:

> The great majority of doctors earned hardly as much as the maintenance of life required. The unequivocal distribution of wealth which was accumulated in the hands of certain families and gave the great masses of the people over to poverty, offered to but few doctors the opportunity of acquiring riches by the exercise of their art. The inconsiderate competition, for which they themselves were responsible, contributed also to this state of affairs by reducing the rate of pay for their services to the smallest possible. Whoever has a poor practice remains necessarily himself a poor man (4).

Outside of Rome proper the lower classes were served, in the main, by communal physicians, who were paid an annual stipend. These physicians, though allowed to carry on private practice, were required to treat the poor without charge. Rome itself had an official regional physician for each district. Also, according to R. Biran, there were numerous physicians attached to distinctive occupational groups, such as the gladiators, circus personnel, and those of the theatre.

The office of *Archiatri populares,* the paid medical officers of the town, writes Puschmann, was very likely maintained in many towns of Italy "from ancient times through the entire period of the middle ages."

> The duties of the town medical officers were—to attend gratis the officials of the town and the poor of the town, to provide medical service for the town hospitals, to assist the magistrates as experts, and to accompany the citizens into the field in time of war; they also exercised control over the apothecaries' shops and licensed houses, and conducted the public sanitary service. At a later period in many places they also undertook the teaching of the lower class of attendants on the sick and examined them.
>
> In Venice, to cite one example, there were 12 physicians and 12 surgeons appointed by the town; the former receiving from 15 to 100 ducats annual pay and the latter from 10 to 130. Even smaller places devoted a regular sum to this purpose in their budget of expenditure. Treviso paid its three public medical officers 728 lire a year, Conegliana 350 lire to physicians, 250 to surgeons, and Palermo paid its two town doctors 50 ounces of gold a year.
>
> In Germany public medical officers were first appointed in the 14th century. In an order of the Emperor Sigismund, of the year 1426, it is said: "In every imperial town there is to be a chief-doctor; he is to be paid 100 gulden."
>
> A church must provide him with them. He is to physic when necessary each and everyone gratis and he must earn his pay by true and faithful service. Frankfort-on-the-Main had in 1348 a town doctor who received clothing and 30 curnocks of corn; there were afterwards three and their pay ranged between 10 and 100 gulden. Doctors were also appointed for the troops, the hospitals, the monasteries, and particular prisons, and received regular pay (5).

It will be gathered, then, that throughout the ages the patterns of medical practice have varied from period to period and from place to place. The physician commonly subscribed to some ethical testament, of which the Oath of Hippocrates was prototypical, and by that pledge was bound to treat his patients decently and humanely. These were his *inner* commitments, the moral framework of his practice. However, how he related in other respects to his patients and they to him depended largely on the given historic time and circumstances, on the given state of cultural, social, economic, and informational development.

Modern medicine is in many respects a derivative of modern socioeconomic developments. Specifically, it was engendered by the growth of cities, by the development of modern commerce and industry, and by the rise and extension of the middle class, of the professional and functionary groups, and of the proletariat. By these eventuations, the "market" for medical service was greatly enlarged, and medicine itself developed a more effective and, hence, more marketable service.

The Middle Ages saw a sprouting of many centers, with dense and spreading populations. It is in these centers, proximate to the universities and hospitals, inspired and animated by the new learning emerging therefrom, and responsive to the needs and demands of the more numerous and wealthy new class of citizen (the bourgeoisie), that the modern patterns of medical practice had their origin. Here the cardinal elements of free choice, fee for service, and the confidential relations of patient and doctor, were crystallized and soon acquired the sanction of established principles. Medical practice, it can be said, developed a mercantilist spirit, the spirit of a "cash nexus." Heretofore, the practice of medicine, was, at least in tradition, a consecration, a devotion to the service of Man, wherein the compensation received was not a reward for that which was given, but only an incident in the business of living. Now it took on the character of a new engagement between patient and physician, involving a *quid pro quo* passed between two personages of equal stature and prerogatives. It was a *free exchange,* and free exchange was the inspiring ideal of the new world of the entrepreneurs, the merchants, bankers, master craftsmen, and nascent industrial capitalists. Medicine, losing none of its idealist heritage, did in effect take on the ideational and practice patterns of the emergent and dominant middle class, the class which directed the rise and attainments of modern Europe.

It is difficult to assign precise dates to the initiation or the culmination of large historical developments. The revolution I have so sketchily presented took place between the 15th and the *end* of the 19th century. This last statement implies that the era of "free exchange" or of the "cash nexus" is now over.

The beginning of its end was marked by the passage of Bismarck's Sickness Insurance Act on June 15, 1883. Yet that "beginning" had a long gestation period, reaching back into the Middle Ages. Social insurance was not a German invention, nor were Bismarck's political motives—to arrest the socialist movement—the sole, the dominant, or the determining reason why the pioneering step in social security legislation was taken in that country. A significant determinant was the fact that Germany was relatively a latecomer among the modern industrial nations. It had to catch up in a hurry. As Sigerist points out:

> Social insurance is a result of the industrialization of the world. In

> the feudal society of the Middle Ages the economically weak individual was the responsibility of his lord or was an object of charity. The idea of mutual insurance took root with the disintegration of feudalism. Already in the late Middle Ages craftsmen's guilds organized mutual benefit funds; the miners, somewhat later, formed brotherhoods that served a similar purpose. When the guilds lost their political power, they nevertheless preserved in many cases their welfare institutions.
>
> The development of capitalism greatly increased the insecurity of the working class, and the situation became very acute in the 19th century, *after* the Industrial Revolution. Millions of people depended on the labor market for a living. Working long hours on wages too low to permit savings, exposed to many hazards, they were thrown out of work by accidents, disease, old age, and by the periodic economic crises that are inherent in capitalist production. Without reserves from which to draw, they become public charges, recipients of a charity that was unable to cope with a problem of such magnitude (6).

Social insurance indubitably is a result of the industrialization of the world. But the dynamics of that result is not entirely summed up in terms of the monetary insecurity and misery of the "working class."

In the last years of the Middle Ages we see a working group emerging which was historically unique—the proletariat—who possessed nothing but their labor power. The reason for the increase of this propertyless class is not that more and more people were deprived of their rightful ownership of the tools for their work—but rather that the new capitalism made it possible for more and more people to survive. Hayek expounds this seeming paradox as follows:

> The actual history of the connection between capitalism and the rise of the proletariat is almost the opposite of that which the theories of the expropriation of the masses suggest. The truth is that, for the greater part of history, for most men the possession of the tools for their work was an essential condition for survival or at least for being able to rear a family. The number of those who could maintain themselves by working for others, although they did not themselves possess the necessary equipment, was limited to a small proportion of the population. The amount of arable land and of tools handed down from one generation to the next limited the total number who could survive. To be left without them meant in most instances death by starvation or at least the impossibility of procreation. There was little incentive and little possibility for one generation to accumulate the additional tools which would have made possible the survival of a larger number of the next, so long as the advantage of employing

> additional hands was limited mainly to the instances where the division of the tasks increased the efficiency of the work of the owner of the tools. It was only when the larger gains from the employment of machinery provided both the means and the opportunity for their investment that what in the past had been a recurring surplus of population doomed to early death was in an increasing measure given the possibility of survival. Numbers [i.e., population] which had been practically stationary for many centuries began to increase rapidly. The proletariat which capitalism can be said to have "created" was thus not a proportion of the population which would have existed without it and which it had degraded to a lower level; it was an additional population which was enabled to grow up by the new opportunities for employment which capitalism provided (7).

This "additional population" added up to a massive increment. Thus the population of England in 1600 is estimated to have numbered 4,460,000; a century later in 1700 it was 5,653,000, and in 1801 it was 8,331,000. Sir Robert Peel in 1806 saw in the Industrial Revolution the mainspring of "an additional race of man" which he credited to the greater "comforts of the population and early marriages."

On this score Sir Robert was an enthusiast. In fact, there was both want and misery, and a great deal of it. This has been amply detailed by the Hammonds in their classic works on the Village and the Town Labourers (8).

The misery of the proletariat inspired much humanitarian concern, which materialized in social legislation and in the Sanitation movement. Society became acutely aware of disease and death, for both were startlingly manifest in the industrial centers: in Boston, London, Birmingham et al. The *Zivilisationsseuche* as the Germans termed them, the "plagues of civilization," the diseases of malnutrition, of overcrowding, of insanitation, of overwork—cholera, tuberculosis, typhus, typhoid, the infant diarrheas, rickets, the pneumonias, scarlet fever, diphtheria—all these were rampant, most intensively among the working class, but also among the middle class.

Thus, with the development of industrialism, the rise of the proletariat, and the concentration of great numbers of human beings in industrial centers, much disease was engendered, and the greater need for medical service of superior competence became manifest and urgent. Hence it can fairly be said that modern medicine derived its sociocultural impulsion from modern industrialism, especially since the beginning of the 19th century.

The consumers of medical services clearly were divisible into two groups—the middle class which provided the bulk of "private practice," and the poorer class, which was served in clinics, and dispensaries, in contract practice, and as charity patients. Many people, of course, were intermediate between these groups; in general, they were treated as if they were of the middle class, but were often charged lower fees.

The extension of the market for medical services is mirrored in the remarkable increase during the 18th and 19th centuries of hospitals, medical schools, and medical personnel. This increase was in quality as well as numbers. "For two-hundred years after the Reformation," wrote Sir Arthur Thomson (9), "England was virtually without hospitals of any kind." "England then was a rural and semi-feudal country; the sick were scattered in villages, and it was not until toward the end of the eighteenth century that the patient was completely and quickly changed by the Industrial Revolution."

"Sickness widely spread in an agricultural community with village workshops might escape notice, but the misery of the sick poor congregated in makeshift towns without sanitation was intensified and compelled attention." "It is not surprising, therefore, that the eighteenth century witnessed the foundation of a large number of charitable institutions in the shape of voluntary hospitals."

The creation of these many hospitals logically increased the demand for medical attendants, and as Sir Arthur observes, "An immediate consequence of the foundation of the new hospitals was the extension of the system of apprenticeship to their wards. The privilege of taking apprentices was a valuable perquisite for the members of the hospital staff. Not only could they exact substantial fees from their pupils but they also obtained free service at negligible costs."

Hospital apprenticeship was an advance over the system of "indentured pupil," by which young men gained their practical experience in medicine, after having "first graduated in arts and become proficient enough in classical scholarship to read Galen and write a commentary in Latin as a thesis for the medical degree."

The growth of the voluntary hospitals stimulated the demand for added instruction and resulted first in the formation of private schools of anatomy, run for profit, and later the establishment of medical schools within the precincts of the hospitals or closely associated with them.

This sketch has been drawn against the background of British experience. But essentially it also represents American experience and practice. American medicine was rooted in British medicine and later also absorbed much of French and German science. However, in respect to its patterns of practice, American medicine was (until very recently) akin to that of British medicine. In addition to the cultural kinship that bound our land with England and its people, there was another and more immediate influence at play. Many of the more earnest American medical aspirants studied and were trained in English and Scottish schools. The latter were the more favored. "John Morgan and William Shippen, who pioneered the College of Philadelphia curriculum in medicine in 1765, were Edinburgh graduates, as were also 112 other Americans by the end of the century. An equal number studied in Edinburgh without receiving the degree. . . . American institutional medical education during the last three and a half decades of the 18th century was extensively influenced by old-world medical education, especially Scottish and English" (10).

Willard C. Rappleye succinctly describes the problems which the nation confronted during the 19th century. "In the rapid expansion of the country the population became widely scattered. Communication and transportation were inadequate and uncertain. Doctors for local communities were needed before the means of educating them were available. With only a few exceptions there were no university opportunities for the study of medicine. . . . There were no hospital facilities for such preparation comparable to those in Great Britain and France. The apprenticeship system was merely expanded to meet the pressing need. Early in the last century less than 10 percent of the physicians in this country were graduates of medical schools. More than 80 percent had never even attended lectures in a school of medicine" (11). Despite the duress of conditions and despite many weaknesses, the profession produced during this period some brilliant educators, men whose names live on in the annals of medical education—John Morgan, William Shippen, David Hosack, the Warrens, Daniel Drake, Nathan Smith. Other competent teachers and a multitude of lesser known medical educators spawned a breed of practitioners not unlike themselves, who in a time of intense nationalism and migrating frontiers, succored a race of men who were dedicated to defense of the rights of the individual and of man's quest for wealth (12).

So much for the emergence of the modern doctor, his education and training. What of those whom he served, and notably of the proletariat, the working class? Much has been written of the latter's hardship, poverty, physical and moral misery, and ill health; and their plight is not to be minimized. True it is, as Kitson Clark says: "What the industrial revolution had provided was the chance of life to men and women who might otherwise have had to face the necessity of death . . . and life, even if your home is a cellar in a Manchester [New York or Boston] slum, was probably better than death by a roadside in Galway, if it was not much better" (12). But the "chance" for many was not "life"; it was little more than survival.

Yet conditions did improve as the 19th century unrolled. The application of science and new techniques to industry, along with methods of mass production, yielded a new way of life. Goods in great variety and massive quantity were produced and the yielded wealth percolated down through the various middle classes until it reached a section of the working class. What at the beginning of the century was largely an amorphous mass of economically and socially disengaged beings became in the latter decades "a new working class, self-conscious, relatively though not extravagantly prosperous, and in a position to stand up for its own rights" (13).

Among the rights it claimed was access to competent medical care. Initially this was affirmed and effected in the patterns of self help, in the formation of trade unions and in the creation of Friendly Societies, Workers Lodges, and Circles. The latter invariably included among their objectives the provision of some forms of medical care, for, as Lord Beveridge repeatedly affirms, "Desire for security in sickness is the original seed from which above all friendly societies have grown."

It is this group, the new working class, the "self-conscious, relatively though not extravagantly prosperous" workers, that has so greatly enlarged the market for medicine, even as the emergent middle class did some centuries before. Of the two, it can now be said that in the more recent decades their lines of demarcation have been fading. They are currently more mergent than distinctive, they tend to form a continuum, not (as Karl Marx prognosticated) by the degradation of the middle class to the level of the proletariat but rather by forming the new conglomerate citizenry of an affluent and socially inspired State.

The enlarged market for medical services profoundly affected the profession. Thus, during the decade following the final enactment of Bismarck's social insurance legislation in 1889, Germany's population increased by a little over 11 percent; but the number of physicians increased by 56 percent.

Great Britain and the United States enacted no sickness insurance schemes between 1890 and 1900, but in these countries, too, the rate of increment in the number of physicians exceeded that of the population. Thus, the population of Britain increased during 1890 to 1900 by 12.8 percent, and the number of physicians by 16.0 percent. In the United States the population increased by 20.7 percent, physicians by 25.9 percent.

No doubt the medical market, so to say, prospered also, because medicine was now in a position to offer more and better service.

My main conclusion is that the patterns of medical practice—i.e., the ways in which the physician serves the patient, in what manner and setting, and in what order of relationship, both contractual and economic—are determined not by the medical profession but by the socioeconomic forces dominant at the given time.

The socioeconomic system at present prevailing throughout the Western sphere has attained such complexity that our patterns of medical practice are no longer entirely suitable or entirely effective. Nor are they always suited to the more complex science and technology of medicine. Both society and science have grown enormously.

This is not an endorsement of what is rather loosely termed Socialized Medicine. It is a simple exposition, based on historic analyses, to show that there are no authentic "sacred cows" among the various forms of medical practice. It is also a plea that we shed our mythic beliefs, and deal with the current reality, realistically.

REFERENCES

1. Puschmann, T. *A History of Medical Education.* London: Lewis, 1891, p. 66.
2. *Ibid.,* p. 67.
3. *Ibid.,* p. 68.
4. Galen, xii, 916. See Puschmann, *Op. cit.,* p. 126.
5. Puschmann, T. *Op. cit.,* pp. 278 and 279.
6. Sigerist, H. *On the History of Medicine.* New York: M.D. Publications, 1960.
7. Hayek, F. A. In: *Capitalism and the Historians.* Chicago: The University of Chicago Press, 1937, p. 15.
8. Hammond, J. L. & B. *The Village Labourer. The Town Labourer.* London: Longmans, 1920.
9. Johnson, A. P. History and development of teaching hospitals in England. *Brit. Med.* J., 1960, ii, 749.
10. Norwood, W. F. American medical education from the Revolutionary War to the Civil War. *J. Med. Educ.,* 1957, 32, pp. 433, 434.
11. Rappleye, W. C. Major changes in medical education during the past fifty years, Feb. 10, 1959.
12. Norwood, W. F. *Op. cit.*
13. Clark, G. K. *Listener.* London: March 16, 1961.

13

The Amateur in Medical History

Clio, who has taken History under her gracious patronage, is one of the nine pulchritudinous daughters of Zeus. Since Clio is a Greek maiden, it is fair to assume that she may be wooed and can be won. She has many admirers and a few suitors. All these can be classed in three groups—the dilettantes, the amateurs, and the cognoscenti. The dilettante flirts with History, the connoisseur is wedded to it, the amateur is its Platonic lover.

To be a true connoisseur of history is a blessing bestowed upon few. A masterly knowledge of history and the competence to cultivate it with profit to the discipline demand first of all a life of labor and devotion and requires, in addition, an intelligence catholic in its encompassment, a sympathy rich in intuitional competences, and more than average talent in languages. Few mortals are so well endowed, and even among these, few are so placed that they can develop their endowments. Perforce, then, most of us must reconcile ourselves to the amateur's status, hoping that in some future life we may be better privileged.

But what is this amateur's status—and how is it to be distinguished from that of the dilettante? The suggestive distinction of flirtation on the part of the dilettante and Platonic love on the part of the amateur is more poetical than instructive or useful. It is necessary, then, to distinguish the two more minutely.

How is the dilettante to be described? We said he flirts with history, with medical history in this instance. The term flirt is a happy one, for it has many connotations, most of which are subsumed in the one—to trifle or to be a trifler. Nothing, to my mind, more aptly describes the essential characteristic of the dilettante. He trifles, he sports, he is, as the dictionary defines him, a superficial amateur. John Brown, in his

Spare Hours (First Series, p. 43), tells of the gruff reply which the painter Opie made to a dilettante who asked him, "What do you mix your colours with?" The retort was, "With brains, Sir!"

More particularly, the dilettante in medical history is not devoted to medical history. It is rather his avocation, a pastime-stuffing for his idle hours. It is unrelated to his life and to his work. It is his accidental hobby, which might as well have been postage stamps or match covers. His products, when he is productive, carry the hallmark of his trifling workshop. Most of his pieces are picayune, even when they are *précieux*. They are incidental, most often trivial. Generally they are unrelated to each other, they reveal no connecting bonds, no reigning motifs. At his best the dilettante polishes pebbles; at his worst he paraphrases the words and thoughts of others, strutting like a playing child in the borrowed clothes of his elders. But that which is amusing in the child is a bore in the dilettante, for the child avowedly plays, while the dilettante expects us to take him in earnest. How many times has one been obliged to listen to the pretentious papers of the dilettante, his every word reminding us of the far superior originals from which by verbal dilution he made his thin gruel?

Enough then, about the dilettante. What now the amateur, how is he to be characterized? His distinguishing mark is his earnestness, which arises out of the compelling love which he bears for medical history. His is not an optative affection, to be put on and off as convenience requires. His love is rather ever with him, for it springs from his everyday need to know and to understand. To the amateur, medical history is not an avocation; on the contrary, it is rooted in his vocation. Get him to confess how he was first smitten, and invariably he will tell you that it was when, in a busy hour, it dawned on him that he was deficient in knowledge and in understanding in some particular of his work. It may have been no more than the realization that Glisson is not the name of a capsule, but rather that of a man, and that the man was unknown to him. It may have been something more weighty. Some curiosity sprung again as an offshoot of the day's work, such as the long time span between the discovery of the microscope and that of the pathogenic organisms. Almost always, however, you will find that it was an intellectual curiosity that led the amateur to become a devotée of Clio. And it is intellectual curiosity, never idle but always pertinent to his life to his work, that holds the amateur in sustained devotion. This is most luminously reflected in the writings of one of the most distinguished amateurs of medical history, William Osler.

For this reason, too, you will find that the amateur's productions, though spotted in many terrains, have a common character and are tied together by his unique interests, by his distinguishing concern. Often they reflect his growing interest and his maturing understanding. Though incidental in their singular content, they tend to form an organic and significant whole in their collective bulk.

There is still another and a most significant hallmark by which the product of the amateur can be distinguished from that of the dilettante, and often, too, from that of the professional medical historian. His works are leavened with his experiences. They are more temporal than the works of the professional, more passionate than those of the dilettante. The reason for this is easy to appreciate, for the works of the amateur drew their motives from troubling necessity, from some urgent problem to which his works, happily, constitute an answer. Like the dilettante, the amateur must borrow from the works of others, but whereas the dilettante borrows like a spendthrift, unmindful of his substance, the amateur borrows so that he may gain a profit by adding his labor to the borrowed capital.

So, much, then, for delineating the characteristics of the amateur in medical history. Now let us observe closely the manner in which he works, the approaches he takes to medical history. They differ somewhat according to his native competence and his experience. During his younger years he is most likely to be interested in simple facts, that is in deeds, actions, performances, discoveries. In the more advanced stage of his development he is bound to discover that behind the facts stand personalities and that facts can better be understood within the framework of the personalities they involve. In his maturity the amateur medical historian strives not only to know, but also to understand. He goes beyond the facts, beyond the actors, and includes in his study the stage setting with all its major elements. It is patent that we have here a scheme of developmental stages and a table of ascending values. I would not have either of these taken too rigorously. On the other hand, I am certain experience will endorse the contention that it is simpler to establish the elmentary facts, those that respond to the queries *who, what, where,* and *when,* than it is to delineate the plays of personality and to gain the answers to the questions *why* and *what is the meaning and significance of it all?*

Illustrative of a problem in elementary facts—who, what, where, and when—is a recent preoccupation of mine with the phrase *Ecclesia abhorret a sanguine*: "the Church abhors blood." You will find this phrase in many medical histories and it is generally credited to the Council of Tours, 1163. It is cited as illustrative of the persecution of surgery by the Church, the degradation of surgery during the Middle Ages being thus accounted for in part.

Now I confess to a deep suspicion that this phrase is spurious; that it is, if you please, a Protestant libel on the Church. I have done some little work on the problem and find no general agreement as to the prohibition implied or the Council, Pope, or Synod that allegedly pronounced the prohibition. Thus far I have not succeeded in finding the phrase employed in any connection in any of the many Councils implicated. I expect to be able to discover who, earliest among the writers of medical history, made this charge and cited the phrase. I shan't be surprised to find him living and writing after the Reformation, and, a Protestant.

Now the mechanics of such a study, you must perceive, are simple though the labor itself may be large. In substance, however, it responds to the queries *who, what, when, where.*

Contrast with this another type of problem, one involving not only certain elementary facts, but also one principal and possibly many related personalities. Consider the problem presented by Mesmer—the father of Mesmerism. The man is portrayed equivocally as charlatan or as martyr. It is not likely that he could have been both; he may have been neither.

To understand the phenomenon of Mesmer and of Mesmerism, it is necessary to take into account his ancestry, the region of his birth and youth, the atmosphere in which he was raised, the teachers he had, the aptitudes he revealed in his early years. It is significant that Mesmer was, in his formative years, a student of Paracelsus, that his mother eagerly desired him to become a priest, that he was very fond of music and had befriended Schumann. His marriage to a wealthy widow, for whom he appears to have had no great affection, is an important facet of his personality. His restlessness is another. Equally vital to the appreciation of Mesmer is a knowledge of the age in which he lived and of the thoughts current in that period. The years of Mesmer were 1734-1815. The world was at this time in an intellectual ferment and grossly materialistic, indeed, mechanistic. The impact of Bacon, Newton, and Descartes was felt as a "terremote" in all domains of thought. Cartesian philosophy, thoroughly mechanistic, exercised as deep an influence on thought in the 17th and 18th centuries as Spencer's *Principles* did on that of the second half of the 19th century. During this period, too, there was much interest in magnetism and electricity. William Gilbert, as will be recalled, published his epoch-making work *De Magnete* in 1600, and set the study of magnetism and of static electricity on a sound foundation. Luigi Galvani, Alessandro Volta, Von Kleist, Benjamin Franklin—men illustrious in the history of electricity—were all contemporaries of Mesmer. All of these factors—the temperament of the man, his early experiences, the mood and intellectual preoccupations of his age—help us to understand Mesmer and Mesmerism.

From this hasty articulation of what is no more than the dry bones of the matter one can perceive how very different a task it is to expound the facts within the framework of the personalities affected than it is to determine what may properly be called the depersonalized facts. It is far more difficult, and yet infinitely more gratifying. The amateur has reached to full rank when he has attained such competence.

There is yet a third approach to medical history open to the amateur. I shall not expound it here, but you can appreciate it readily by compounding and multiplying the second approach until it embraces the many personalities and events that form an epoch. The problems treated are of an interpretative nature, responding to the questions *why,* and *what does it mean?* Why was the medicine of the 18th century dominated by the system builders? What bearing has the rise of clinical psychiatry during the last two centuries upon the contemporaneous agnosticism and atheism?

The approaches to medical history, like the roads to Rome, are many. I have designated for the amateur three broad avenues, some level, some steep. I have written, perhaps more disparagingly than is warranted, of dilettantism in medical history. I can only end with a prayer of thanks to the lovely Clio, daughter of Zeus, patron of our devotion. May it be given us long to enjoy her favor so that our labors may be more fruitful, and may our understanding grow with our years.

14

On the "Futility" of Medical History

The wise and worldly H. L. Mencken, famed as the "Sage of Baltimore," lists in his *Dictionary of Quotations on Historical Principles from Ancient and Modern Sources* no fewer than 93 quotations dealing with history *per se.* These are drawn from a host of sources ranging from Genesis, Thucydides and Polybius, to Karl Marx, Henry Ford and that most prolific of all authors, the Unidentified One. Incidentally, his is the smartest of all definitions of history. "History," the Unidentified One said, "is something that never happened, written by a man who wasn't there." That definition is worth ruminating, for even if it *did happen,* more often than not it didn't happen the way the man who wasn't there describes it.

Mr. Mencken was prone to write with tongue in cheek; hence one suspects him of a cynical bias when, in scanning his selected quotations, one finds the majority casting doubt on the veracity and worth of history as it is told. "I am ashamed to see what a shallow village tale our so-called history is," wrote Ralph Waldo Emerson. Ambrose Bierce saw in history "an account mostly false, of events unimportant, which are brought about by rulers mostly knaves, and soldiers mostly fools." Herbert Spencer defined history as "the masses of worthless gossip furnished us by historians." The authors quoted who did not utterly disbelieve the tales told by historians saw in history a parade of human misery, cruelty and stupidity. Edward Gibbon saw history as "little more than the register of the crimes, follies and misfortunes of mankind," and Voltaire viewed it as "only a picture of crimes and misfortunes."

Only the very ancient authors, and in modern times the German philosophers, have had a strong faith in the tutorial values of history. It was Thucydides who foisted on us the misleading persuasion that history repeats itself, a persuasion which with some radical modifications was adopted by the German philosopher, Hegel. If history does indeed repeat itself, then the past is not, as we now believe, merely a prelude to the future, but is rather the youthful image of aging experience. Cicero grandiloquently spoke of history as "the witness of the times, the torch of truth, the life of memory, the teacher of life, the messenger of antiquity." "History is a philosophy teaching by examples," wrote Dionysius of Halicarnassus. These few sentiments and opinions were shared by a few moderns. Freud, for example, saw in history "a voice forever sounding across the centuries the laws of right and wrong." Hegel was fully persuaded that history had much to teach us, but wrote that "Peoples and government have never learned anything from history, or acted on principles deducible from it."

The ancients were, or so it would seem, rather naive and the moderns far too romantic. We cannot entirely subscribe to the opinion ascribed to Henry Ford that "history is bunk," yet we are persuaded that much history, as it is commonly and widely written and taught, is futile and this applies most notably to *medical* history. For the writing and teaching of general history has been subjected during the past hundred years to sharp scrutiny and thoroughgoing criticism. As a result it has been largely freed of naivete and purged of romanticism.

Karl Marx claimed to have set Hegel on his head by substituting economic determinism for the Hegelian thesis that history moving in spiral circuits mirrors "the development of freedom, which is identical with the moral reason of man as exhibited in an external system of social relations" (1). Subsequently, both Hegel and Marx were, so they say, taken apart by Croce, Ortega y Gasset, Dilthey and Collingwood. A masterful critique of the philosophy of history which sees in history the unravelment of purpose, which pretends to discern in the evolution of history rhythms, patterns, laws and trends, is to be found in Karl Popper's book, *The Poverty of Historicism* (2). Its dedication, incidentally, is most noteworthy, for it is inscribed to the memory of the countless men and women of all creeds, nations and races who fell victim to the fascist and communist belief in the inexorable laws of historical destiny.

While the study, writing and teaching of general history, as noted, has been critically analyzed and re-examined with much profit and good effects, that of medical history has in the main remained backward, if not archaic. I have in mind particularly the academic works and teachings of the official university departments of medical history. Telling contributions have been made by some few, non-academic students of medical history and these are not to be included in this extended criticism. But they are few, and the academicians do not always approve of or encourage their labors.

The essential deficiencies in academic medical history derive from its commitment to the "great man, great discoveries" view of medical history and of medical progress. It chronicles the tales of *the* medical heroes, *their* wars against ignorance and disease, *their* conquests. In the persuasion pronounced by Thomas Carlyle, himself a hero worshipper, that "universal history is at bottom the history of the great men who have worked here," the academicians grub among the chronicles and leavings of the great, ad nauseam, and count it the attainment of earnest scholarship when they have signaled an overlooked edition, a heretofore unnoticed variation in a reading, or the forerunner of a celebrated observation. Assuredly these *are* among the useful, even if trivial, data of medical history, but those who labor long at such gathering are prone to mistake their miscellany of accumulations for real knowledge and deep understanding. It were not so bad if the academicians were content to grub and would suffer others without molestation to cultivate the *understanding* of medical history. But that lies not in the nature of the creature which, because of its myopic intelligence, its utter dependence upon the *already* published word, becomes panicky in the presence of judgment, opinion and understanding, unbuttressed by the apparatus of citations, quotations and references. The academicians do not understand that originality creates the occasion for citations and references but does not rest upon them.

Friedrich von Schiller, poet and historian, acutely observed and described these qualities of the academicians, whom he tellingly labeled the *Brotgelehrte.** He wrote, "Every extension of his pedestrian lore (*Brotwissenschaft*) makes him anxious, for it either commits him to new labors or renders his past ones useless. Every significant innovation frightens him, for it disrupts the old patterns of thought which he had so laboriously structured, and menaces him with the loss of his life's work." "Every light sparked in whatever field of knowledge by fortuitous genius makes patent the inadequacies of the *Brotgelehrte* (hacks of learning). They fight with bitterness, with malice, despondently, for in defense of their school of thought they at the same time fend for their total being" (3).

* A literary hack, one who is obliged to live by his learning, or who turns to learning for the sake of gaining his substance.

But there is little sport in hunting them down. They are the pale, bloodless devotees of the philosophy of the great men and of the great discoveries. It is the philosophy that is at fault.

This philosophy is clearly expounded in Fielding H. Garrison's preface to Sir William Osler's *The Evolution of Modern Medicine* (4). "Osler," he wrote, "saw clearly and felt deeply that the men who have made an idea or discovery viable and valuable to humanity are the deserving men; he has made the great names shine out, without depreciation of the important work of lesser men . . ."

Implicit in the "great men, great discoveries" philosophy of medical history and of medical progress is the assumption that medicine is an evolving science whose progression is animated by its own innate forces and whose direction is determined by its own inherent logic. The progress of medicine is represented as an accretive process wherein, with passing time, fact is added to fact, knowledge is summated in mounting totals, and truth becomes ever more refined. It also presumes the fortuitous and providential advent of good men with great minds capable of conceiving "the truth," albeit piecemeal.

In effect, however, there is no golden thread that runs consecutively and continuously throughout the history of medicine. The progress of medicine does not follow a pattern logically consistent with its own historical antecedents. Medical progress is more episodic than orderly or logical. Medicine is not an autonomous, self-animating and self-directing science and discipline. Medicine is shaped by the cultural forces that impinge upon it at any given historical period. Medicine is inspired, animated and directed by a host of determinate forces deriving from the existent and specific geographic, economic, technological, political and ethical factors.

Henry Sigerist well appreciated all this. "The history of medicine," he wrote, "is both history and medicine. It is one aspect of the history of civilization and part of the theory of medicine. . . . When you pursue your historical studies into the present, you imperceptibly enter the field of sociology and begin to see that an infinite number of non (medical) scientific factors—social, economic, political, philosophical, religious—may well determine success or faliure of medicine, factors which must be investigated" (5).

In the pursuit of these convictions Sigerist planned to develop the Hopkins Institute of Medical History so that it would embrace two divisions, one of the history of medicine and the other of the sociology and economics of medicine. His plan fell through, largely because, as

Sigerist phrased it, "it was impossible to find the money, not only on account of the depression, but chiefly because the subject is one that might easily yield controversial results." Sigerist did not say precisely what those controversial results might be, but among them, as I can attest from personal experience and observation was the very issue expounded here—to wit, that medicine, and hence its history, is shaped by the social, economic, technological, political and ethical factors that impinge upon it at the given historical period. Sigerist was criticized and disparaged for venturing into these perimeter fields. He was deemed the less pure, and the less authentic a medical historian, for doing so. But his memory and reputation are in the safekeeping of time.

Medicine is now deeply involved in the great revolution that signals the emergence of a new society—a society that is committed to social welfare and that confronts the challenge of affluence in material means and in leisure time. Medicine not only needs to learn how best to meet the service requirements of this new Society of the Common Man but must also be prepared to participate in its effective development.

For each of these tasks we are ill prepared. For during the greater portion of medicine's long history, most of its practitioners were literally in the service of the rich and the powerful; and during the more recent centuries, most have mainly served the middle class. Granted that the doctor was also a Good Samaritan and often looked after the poor for little or no payment, his historic orientation has been with, and that of, the uncommon, rather than the common man. The mordant and revealing jest is that of the prosperous physician who says to the impoverished and sickly patient, "My dear fellow, what you really need is a restful vacation in the country." Those, who, like Johann Peter Frank, were stirred with concern for the health of the masses, were few in number, and until recent times were not very effective in converting their concern into effective action.

Our historic orientation has involved us in many biases; it has entangled us in numerous prejudices, myths and misunderstandings. To set things aright, we need not only to learn much that is new, but also to unlearn much that is old and in error. We need to free ourselves from such encumbrances, we need to reassess our understanding of the history of medicine and of man's medical experiences down the ages. For that, perhaps the very first requisite is that we should shed the conceits which prompt us to believe that we are so much better and wiser than those who preceded us. We are assuredly more knowledgeable, but it is more than likely that in the framework of their given world our elders were relatively as knowledgeable, and possibly even wiser. It were well to be mindful of the Hippocratic injunction, given in his *Ancient Medicine,* "that we ought not to reject the ancient art as non-existent, or on the ground that its method of inquiry is faulty, just because it has not attained exactness in every detail, but rather, because it has been able by reasoning to rise from deep ignorance to approximate perfect accuracy, I think we ought to admire the discoveries as the work not of chance, but of inquiry rightly and correctly conducted" (6)! To this I would add the following quotation from the same book: "I am at a loss to understand how those who maintain the other view, and abandon the old method to rest the art on a postulate, treat their patients on the lines of their postulates. For they have not discovered, I think, an absolute hot or cold, dry or moist, that participates in no other form."

The last affirmation, "They have not discovered the absolute hot or cold," is of profound significance and strikes at the core of the conceit fostered by the academic version of medical history. Pasteur is celebrated for his discovery of the microbic agents of infectious diseases, and Koch shares in these honors. It is taught that the tubercle bacillus is *the cause* of tuberculosis, the typhoid bacillus of typhoid, and so on. But as has been shown a thousand times over, it is *not* true, it is *not* correct. "They have not discovered the absolute hot or cold." Only the negative version has been proved, to wit, "without the tubercle bacillus there can be no tuberculosis," and so on.

I find greater good sense in the Hippocratic version of the *crasis* of hot and cold, dry and moist. For in an agrarian economy, what is more perceptibly determinate for good than just the right and seasonal balance between hot and cold, moist and dry. Excesses in any factor adversely affect crops, and derivatively, beast, bird and man. And as is written in the Hippocratic book *Peri trophees,* the "Power of nutriment reaches to bone and to all parts of bone, to sinew, to vein, to artery, to muscle, to membrane, to flesh, fat and blood, phlegm, marrow, brain, spinal marrow, the intestines and all their parts; it reaches also to heat, breath, and nurture" (7). Here lies a lesson which, alas, many contemporary physicians have yet to learn.

One of the gloomiest chapters in medical history is that devoted to the story of the anticontagionists. These are the men who were unwilling to accept the version of disease causation which credited all pathogenic dynamics to the contagious agent. They have been pilloried, in general, as reactionaries, as ignorant and stubborn men, who stood athwart the path of progress. But many of them were, in effect, not ignorant but rather broadly experienced and widely informed. Many, too, did not deny the pathogenic powers of bacteria, but only the claims of the contagionists that represented the bacteria as the ultimate and determinate agents of disease. Among the anticontagionists there were men who understood the meaning of "epidemic constitution," and who were ecologists (Pettenkofer, for one) even before the term was coined. How little understanding have our academicians had of the historic significance of crowding in relation to the crowd diseases! One searches in vain for the names of Major Greenwood and Sir William Hamer in the indices of the definitive histories of medicine. They are not to be found even in the latest editions, yet these were two of our more preeminent epidemiologists. Greenwood wrote with deep historic and epidemiological insight on the crowd diseases, and Hamer (8) scanned with broad historical understanding the different approaches to the study of diseases and epidemics. Both Greenwood and Hamer (Greenwood the more so) are pungent critics of medicine "as is." They are, therefore, not in style. They do not subscribe to the simple vision of medical progress as a conquest of diseases. They argue, as did in a sense Sydenham, that diseases may be conquered, yet ill health prevail.

And this touches on the very nub of the objection to the "great men, great discoveries" version of medical history, in that this version masks the real essence of medical progress which lies less in the conquest of disease than in the promotion of well being. The anticipation that science will "conquer" disease to the extent that man may in time live his life relatively diseaseless is, as René Dubos has argued, a mirage. I have myself described contemporary medical progress as "a conversion of mortality into morbidity." That I may not be misunderstood, let me here affirm that I am fully in favor of, and prize for myself and for mankind, the "conquering" of diseases by any and all means available, surgery, vaccines, antibiotics, etc. But all that, so much the produce of "great men, making great discoveries," is not the essence of medical progress, our medical histories to the contrary notwithstanding.

The mortality rate from tuberculosis began to decline a half century or more before the tubercle bacillus was discovered and sanatorium treatment was developed. A host of other diseases likewise declined in prevalence, beginning at about the same period, that is, in the first quarter of the 19th century. At about that time, sanctions against unions were lifted both in England and in the United States, and life for most persons, and in particular for the poor, the workers, and women and children, began to improve. Abuses were to some extent curbed by legislation. The public's conscience was aroused and a keener sense of social responsibility engendered. But most significant of all was the mounting "pay-off" of the industrial system. Work became more productive, work hours shorter, real wages higher. Foods that were heretofore scarce and costly became available to the masses: meat and milk and fruit. It all came about slowly, painfully and not without strife. But it did come about. There emerged a new working class which was self-conscious, comparatively prosperous, and able to stand up for its rights—the class that bulks large in the new society.

We need to understand this new society and its needs, medical, psychological, and social. Such understanding is to be gained not by contemplation but by interaction, and in this we need historic perspective, aft and forward. The past is to be reassessed, the present correctly gauged, and the future intelligently projected.

And here we return to medical history. As it has been written, in the pattern of "the great man, great discoveries," it is largely futile. It may entertain, as does good fiction, but it will not serve our needs. We need *that* order of historical study which illuminates the interactions between medicine and the prevailing sociocultural forces, economic, technical, sociologic, moral, and philosophical. Clearly, the academic medical historian is ill equipped to initiate and to develop such studies. Even if he were receptive, he would need the cooperation of other disciplines—economics, sociology, anthropology, general history, and others. As a recluse-grubber, he is not receptive, and hence had better be left alone. What is wanted, then, is what Sigerist had dreamt of, a university-housed institute of social and historical medicine that would embrace the various specialty disciplines.

I am in earnest, and I see ahead of us not a "medical millenium" but a very great challenge, the challenge of medically serving vast numbers of human beings in *new* ways as well as in *old* ways, not only practicing what I have termed episodic (curative) medicine, but also maintenance (physiological or eubiotic) medicine. To practice these orders of medicine it will be necessary that we understand in depth what we are involved in, its derivations, and its issues. For this we need historic knowledge, and historic perspective. We cannot profit by the naive history written in terms of the "great man, great discovery." We need a new order of medical history, one that views medicine as an integral part of the complex of social, technologic and cultural existence.

And the moral is that medical history is too important a subject to leave entirely in the hands of the academic historians.

REFERENCES

1. COLLINGWOOD, R. G. *The Idea of History*. Oxford: Clarendon Press, 1946, p. 114.
2. POPPER, K. R. *The Poverty of Historicism*. Boston: Bean, 1957.
3. VON SCHILLER, F. *Historische Schriften*. Leipzig, Inselverlag, 1906, p. 716.
4. OSLER, W. *The Evolution of Modern Medicine*. New Haven: Yale University Press, 1921, p. xiv.
5. SIGERIST, H. *On the History of Medicine*. New York: M. D. Publications, 1960, p. 245.
6. JONES, W. H. S. *Hippocrates*. New York: Putnam, 1923, vol. i, p. 33.
7. *Ibid.*, p. 345.
8. HAMER, W. *Epidemiology Old and New*. London: Kegan Paul, 1928.

Index